D1716108

An Atlas of Critical Care Chest Roentgenography

Contributors

Diane E. Agin

James I. Breckenfeld, MD

Harley V. Koons, RT

Elias M. Mendoza, MD

Fred Michaelson, RT

Allen J. Stone, MD

Lyle D. Victor, MD

Malcolm L. Weckstein, MD

David Yates, MD

An Atlas of Critical Care Chest Roentgenography

Lyle D. Victor, M.D., F.A.C.P., F.C.C.P.
Director, Pulmonary Disease Section
Oakwood Hospital
Dearborn, Michigan

Radiography Editor
Allen J. Stone, M.D.
Staff Radiologist, Oakwood Hospital

Photography Editor
Michael P. Sarnacki, M.A.
Director, Audio Visual Services
Oakwood Hospital

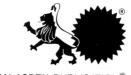

AN ASPEN PUBLICATION®
Aspen Systems Corporation
Rockville, Maryland
Royal Tunbridge Wells
1985

Library of Congress Cataloging in Publication Data

Victor, Lyle D.
An atlas of critical care chest roentgenography.

"An Aspen publication."
Includes bibliographies and index.
1. Chest—Radiography—Atlases. 2. Chest—Diseases—Diagnosis—Atlases. 3. Critical
care medicine—Atlases. 4. Diagnosis, Radioscopic—Atlases. I. Title. [DNLM: 1.
Critical Care—atlases. 2. Thoracic Radiography—atlases. WF 17 V643a]
RC941.V48   1985   617.540757   84-28242
ISBN: 0-87189-076-3

Managing Editor: M. Eileen Higgins
Editorial Services: Scott Ballotin
Printing and Manufacturing: Paul Carlin

The authors and publisher have made every effort to ensure the accuracy of the information herein, particularly with regard to drug selection and dose. However, ap-
propriate information sources should be consulted, especially for new or unfamiliar
drugs or procedures. It is the responsibility of every practitioner to evaluate the ap-
propriateness of a particular opinion in the context of actual clinical situations and
with due consideration to new developments. Authors, editors, and the publisher cannot
be held responsible for any typographical or other errors found in this book.

Library of Congress Catalog Card Number: 84-28262
ISBN: 0-87189-076-3

Printed in the United States of America

1 2 3 4 5

To my twin daughters,
Natalie and Nadine

to Andrew D. Hunt, Jr., MD
Dean of the College of Human Medicine
Michigan State University
1964—1977

whose encouragement of creative effort inspired
my medical writing

Contributors of Roentgenograms

Reza Abghari, MD

Jeffrey Arnold, MD

Lawrence Campbell, MD

Phillip Cascade, MD

Nancy Cardenas, MD

Kyriakos Demetropoulos, MD

Allan Dobzyniak, MD

George Hnatiuk, MD

Howard Kaplan, MD

William Keating, MD

Joon Kie Kim, MD

Thomas Kwyer, MD

Nicholas Lekas, MD

Heront Marcarian, MD

William McDonald, MD

John C. McMicham, PhD

Duane Mezwa, MD

Steven Morse, DD

Pinnamaneni Prasad, MD

Cheryl Sangster, MD

Enrique Signori, MD

Oscar Signori, MD

Technical Credits

Vita Fanders, RT (R)

Harley Koons, RT (R)

Kevin Maycock, RT (R)

Fred Michaelson, RT (R) ARRT

Susan Weinmann, RT (R)

File Room—Oakwood Hospital

Randy Harris

Rob Jablonski

Mark Jakovac

Kathleen Keer

Joe Kozma

Arlene Nicholas

Gary Parker

Michael Washington

Secretaries—Oakwood Hospital

Donna Hernandez

Barbara Richards

Pam Wembam

Library Staff—Oakwood Hospital

Lorraine Obrzut

Joanne Perchall

Sharon Phillips

Phyllis Young

Table of Contents

Foreword

Rapid advances in critical care medicine and the application of new technology for physiologic monitoring have led to improved diagnosis and to better overall management. Although invasive procedures have provided major changes in the way that clinical care is given, they are not without their hazards, and, indeed, on occasion may contribute to the array of complications that already are the lot of the ICU patient. While it is unthinkable that we could manage critically ill patients without new high tech procedures, it is equally true that we must be aware of the problems that these procedures produce. Thus, we have highly important intrinsic complications of the patient's disease and/or surgical operation that are appropriately diagnosed by angiography, CT, and isotope scans, monitored with catheters and tubes; but each invasive system adds another potential iatrogenic set of complications.

Dr. Lyle Victor and his colleagues have summarized their experiences in radiologic evaluation of critically ill patients in this work. While their primary purpose is to illustrate examples of commonly encountered problems, their work also is a useful resource for students, residents, and busy practitioners who wish a concise review of the essential x-ray patterns.

William C. Shoemaker, M.D.

Preface

Rapid technical advances in cardiorespiratory support and hemodynamic monitoring have generated many new chest roentgenographic patterns, which are seen in the critical care patient. A misplaced endotracheal tube or central catheter, pneumothorax, atelectasis, and acute pulmonary edema are complications that can be diagnosed roentgenographically—a procedure that enables clinicians to improve patient care and to save lives. Critical care specialists, house officers, nurses, and respiratory therapists have responsibilities in the interpretation of these acute roentgenographic changes in the critical pulmonary patient.

An Atlas of Critical Care Chest Roentgenography provides, pictorially, the basics of chest radiograph interpretation and the major features of acute chest roentgenography as they are seen in the intensive care unit. (For easy reference, all figures are grouped at the end of the chapters in which they are described.) Intended to provide visually the commonly seen roentgenographic patterns and the regional pathology of both intrinsic and iatrogenic disease, the book may be used as a resource for visual comparison when unfamiliar roentgenographic patterns are encountered on the chest film.

To improve the clinician's ability to do this, the chapters have two general themes about pathological development: (1) pattern recognition, as seen in the chapters on airspace disease, abnormal air and fluid, and catheters and tubes, and (2) regional pathology, as seen in the chapters on cardiovascular disease, complications of intubation and tracheostomy, trauma and surgery, and the critical abdomen. This approach allows for easier reference when viewing unknown roentgenographic pathology. The chapter on neonatal chest roentgenography provides a much needed reference in an area of increasing clinical concern.

A note of special thanks goes to Robert A. Songe, M.D., Chief, Department of Radiology at Oakwood Hospital in Dearborn, Michigan, and to Alan T. Hennessey, M.D., Vice-Chief, Department of Radiology at Oakwood. Their encouragement and assistance made this book possible.

LYLE D. VICTOR, MD, FACP, FCCP

Chapter 1

Roentgenographic Anatomy

Lyle D. Victor, MD, *and Diane E. Agin*

Interpretation of abnormal x-ray films requires knowledge of normal human anatomy. Because the chest roentgenograph provides a two-dimensional representation of the density of three-dimensional structures, it is important that medical personnel have an understanding of normal anatomical spatial relationships. Figures 1–1 and 1–2 are intended to help them gain that understanding.

THE RESPIRATORY PUMP

The human respiratory apparatus is surrounded by bony support. The anteriorly placed clavicles border the lung apices, while the scapulas bound posteriorly, and the sternum, anteriorly. Surrounding the lungs in a circular fashion are the ribs. The inferior border is the thin, muscular diaphragm—the principal muscle of respiration.

The bony framework and the muscles work in concert during inspiration and expiration. Responsible for about 65% of tidal volume, the diaphragm is the most important respiratory muscle (Fig. 1–1). The muscle is thin and dome-shaped, its contour is influenced by the placement of the liver (right inferior), the spleen and stomach (left inferior), and by the right and left lower lobes of the lungs (superior).

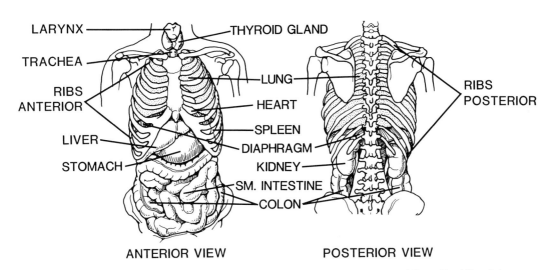

Figure 1–1. Thoraco-abdominal anatomy. Adapted from drawings, courtesy of Henry Ford Hospital.

FISSURES, LOBES, AND SEGMENTS

Lobes and segments are surrounded by connective tissue sacs that are called fissures when viewed from the front (Fig. 1–2). The horizontal fissure separates the right upper lobe from the right lower lobe and is seen best when viewed in an anterior or posterior position. The oblique fissure travels posteriorly or anteriorly in a diagonal direction and is best seen in the lateral view.

A porous structure made up of air, alveolar epithelium, and connective tissue, the lung is penetrated by the branching tracheobronchial tree. The right lung is slightly larger than the left and is subdivided into three lobes and ten segments. The smaller left lung has two lobes and eight segments. Inasmuch as pneumonia, atelectasis, and pulmonary embolae frequently follow a segmental distribution, an understanding of segmental anatomy is clinically useful.

Anterior, lateral, and posterior views of lobes and segments are shown in Figures 1–3 and 1–4.

The right upper lobe has apical, anterior, and posterior segments. The middle lobe has a medial and a lateral segment, and the lower lobe has superior (apical), medial, anterior, lateral, and posterior basal segments. In contrast to its counterpart on the right side, the left upper lobe is a compact unit; it has a combined apical–posterior segment and a lingular lobe composed of superior and inferior segments. The lingular division of the left upper lobe is analogous to the middle lobe on the right. The left lower lobe has a combined anterior-medial segment and lateral and posterior segments.

THE TRACHEOBRONCHIAL TREE

The conduits in gas exchange are the trachea and the branching network of the bronchial tree. These structures appear more prominently on the chest x-ray film because of the increased density from cartilaginous structure. The trachea, a

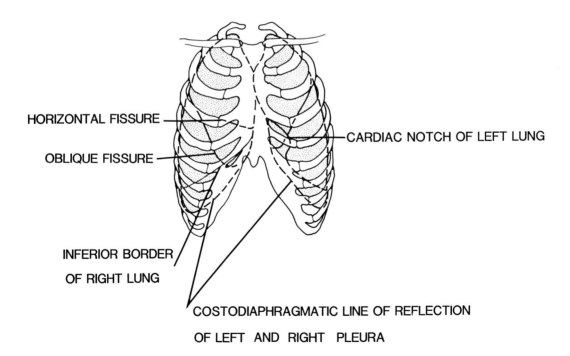

Figure 1–2. Fissures, lobes, and segments. Adapted from drawings, courtesy of Henry Ford Hospital.

LOBES AND SEGMENTS
Posterior and Lateral Views

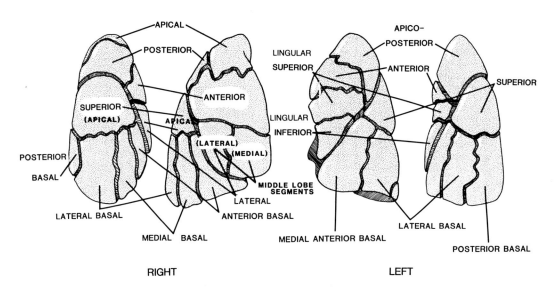

RIGHT

LEFT

Figure 1–3. Lobes and segments: posterior view. Adapted from drawings, courtesy of Henry Ford Hospital.

LOBES AND SEGMENTS:
ANTERIOR VIEW

Right   Left

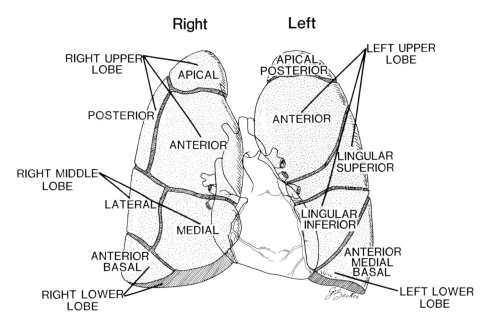

Figure 1–4. Lobes and segments: anterior view. Adapted from drawings, courtesy of Henry Ford Hospital.

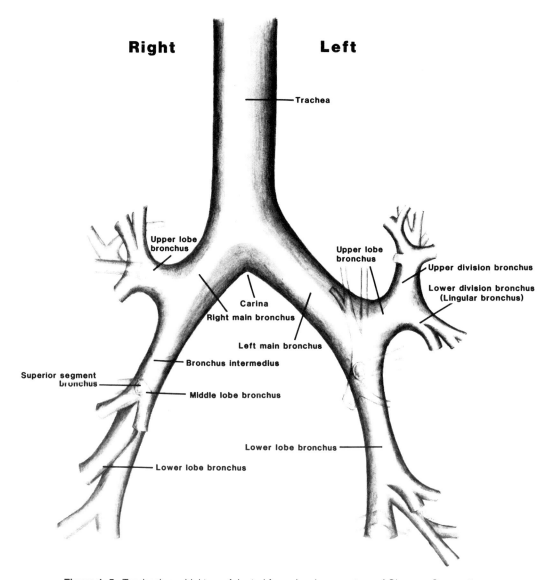

Figure 1–5. Tracheobronchial tree. Adapted from drawing, courtesy of Olympus Corporation.

cylindrical body, begins below the vocal cords, then is surrounded by the thyroid gland, and terminates at the keellike bifurcation of the trachea into the left and right mainstem bronchi known as the carina (Fig.1–5). The left mainstem bronchus angles obliquely off the trachea and divides into the left upper lingular division and the left lower lobe bronchi. The right mainstem bronchus travels inferiorly in a more direct way, dividing into the right upper, the middle, and the lower lobe bronchi.

THE MEDIASTINUM

The mediastinum, an anatomical structure in the middle of the thorax, is composed of the heart, the great vessels, and the lymphatics (Fig. 1–6). Bordered superiorly by the thoracic outlet, medially by the lungs, inferiorly by the diaphragm, anteriorly by the sternum, and posteriorly by the spine, the mediastinum contains the following structures: the trachea, the aorta, the pulmonary arteries (which form the pulmo-

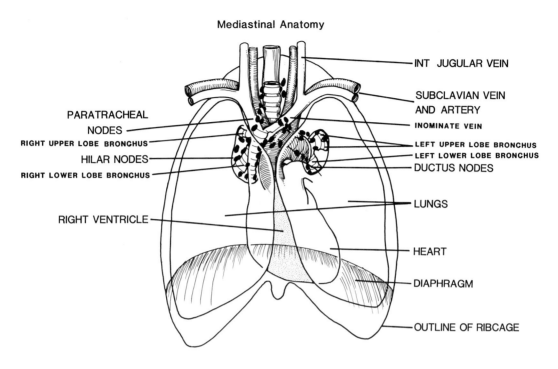

Figure 1–6. Mediastinal anatomy.

nary hilum), the pulmonary veins, the hilar lymph nodes, and the heart. The lungs per se are not part of the mediastinum, although pleural reflections form the lateral border of the mediastinum.

The clinician's understanding of mediastinal anatomy can be critically important because a widening mediastinum can be seen in dissecting thoracic aneurysm, in cases of mediastinitis, and in other acute life-threatening disorders.

Chapter 2

Fundamentals

Fred Michaelson, RT, *Harley V. Koons*, RT,
Malcolm L. Weckstein, MD, *and Lyle D. Victor*, MD

Roentgenology is that branch of medicine dealing with the use of roentgen rays (x-rays) in the diagnosis and treatment of disease. Roentgenography or radiography deals specifically with the art and science of recording x-ray images on photographic film.

A basic understanding of roentgenographic principles should aid critical care personnel in evaluating the adequacy of radiographic technique.

RADIATION PHYSICS

On November 8, 1895, a German physicist, Wilhelm Konrad Roentgen, while observing high voltage discharges in a vacuum cathode tube, discovered the fluorescence of a screen coated with barium platinocyanide located several feet from the cathode tube. He soon realized that this mysterious new ray had the properties to produce a visible impression after penetrating cloth, wood, metal, or human flesh.

Using the mathematical symbol X for the unknown quantity, he called this invisible, penetrating radiation the *x*-ray. Within the next few months, Roentgen further defined the major properties of x-rays and the conditions necessary for their production. In summary, they are the following:

- X-rays are produced whenever high-speed electrons undergo a sudden deceleration, such as striking a metal target in a vacuum tube.

- X-rays cause the fluorescence of certain phosphors and sensitize photographic film, which can then be developed chemically.

- X-rays produce biological and chemical changes in organisms.

In 1901, Roentgen was awarded the first Nobel Prize for Physics for his great discovery, and the x-ray is now linked directly to his name as "Roentgen rays."

Figure 2–1 displays the electromagnetic spectrum of the various kinds of radiant energy. The chart shows that x-rays, located above the visible light spectrum, are of a very high frequency but relatively short wavelength. They also travel at the same constant speed as does light in a vacuum or air and are completely invisible. These physical properties allow x-rays to penetrate tissue and to activate special photographic film to produce an x-ray image or radiograph.

The x-ray cassette is a device used to enhance the reproduction of the radiographic image. It is generally composed of two fluorescent screens superimposed over silver-impregnated photographic film. The patient is placed between the cassette (a film holder and intensifying screen system) and the x-ray beam source (Fig. 2–2). When x-rays penetrate the tissue, they activate the fluorescent screen to emit visible light that causes precipitation of the silver contained in the x-ray film emulsion, in much the same way that photographic film is activated by light in a camera.

FACTORS AFFECTING EXPOSURE

Density and Tissue Thickness

Density and tissue thickness are factors that determine the level of x-ray that can penetrate a subject to activate the intensifying screen(s). Because air in the lungs, for example, causes low tissue density, it allows greater x-ray penetration and causes more precipitation of silver on the film; the result is a dark image on the radiograph. Bone is denser and so allows penetration of fewer x-rays, which results in little activation of the photographic emulsion; the result is a less exposed film. Figure 2–3, a radiograph of a glass bottle filled with air, fat, water, and bone, demonstrates the various densities of human tissue. Air appears darkest radiographically, because it allows the maximum penetration of x-rays. Fat, an intermediate human density, affords more absorption of the x-ray photon and less production of photographic density. Because water and soft tissue are of about the same atomic density, they easily blend together around the finger. Bone is the most dense item represented in this example, and so it allows less x-ray penetration.

Just as density affects radiographic imaging, so does a substance's thickness. Figure 2–4A is a photograph of a step wedge—a metal bar with graduated thickness—used for checking radiographic technique. Figure 2–4B is an x-ray photograph of the bar. Notice that level *a,* the thickest part of the bar, absorbed much of the x-ray beam, leaving the x-ray film relatively inactivated and with less density (white); whereas at level *b,* the metal is much thinner and allowed a greater proportion of the x-ray beam to pass through to activate the film and to produce a dark image.

Kilovoltage and Milliamperage

Density and tissue thickness are not the only factors that affect image intensity. The quantity and the quality of x-radiation produced during a specific time also have their effect.

The quantity of kilovoltage used in chest roentgenography gives an indication of the amount of force or energy contained in the x-ray beam. The greater the energy, the greater is the x-ray's ability to penetrate tissue. This greater energy (kilovoltage) produces a longer scale of contrast. The concept of scale of contrast is depicted in Figures 2–5A and 2–5B, which show two roentgenograms of a 25-cent piece. Figure 2–5A has been taken at low kilovoltage and has a low scale of contrast; that is, the range of densities in the roentgenogram is short, and so there is a large change in tonal value from one density to another, which makes Washington's image unrecognizable. Higher kilovoltage results in long-scale contrast, which makes possible the visualization in a single roentgenogram of a wide range of tissues with different absorption efficiencies. Because the shorter wave length energy afforded by higher kilovoltages allows greater penetration of tissues, it results in an abundance of radiation of varying intensities and, in turn, produces a larger number of tones. The higher kilovoltage used in Figure 2–5B thus generates the multiple tones allowing detailed visualization of the first president's image.

Just as the ampere unit denotes the amount of electricity, it may also represent the quantity of x-rays produced. The milliampere-second (MAS) is the common term used to represent the amount of x-rays delivered per unit of time. Increasing the MAS improves distinctness between densities. However, the amount of tissue damage related to the x-ray exposure is primarily related to the number of x-rays absorbed rather than to their energy. Therefore, it is better roentgenographic technique to get maximum tissue discrimination with higher kilovoltages rather than with higher MAS.

EFFECT OF ROENTGENOGRAPHIC POSITIONING AND TECHNIQUE ON QUALITY

Chest radiography performed in the hospital's x-ray department is ideally done with the patient standing erect, his breath held upon deep inspiration, and the film cassette positioned frontally. The x-ray machines are stationary and powerful, able to generate in excess of 120 kV and several hundred MAS, which allows adequate penetration of the thickest tissue planes. Nevertheless, critical care chest roentgenography has several limitations that affect the quality of imaging. Three of the most significant limitations are (1) low power, (2) positioning, and (3) patient respirations.

Low power mobile units can generate only about 80 kV of energy. It is difficult, therefore, to penetrate thick anatomical parts or to produce diagnostic lateral chest radiographs.

Positioning limitations are presented by critically ill patients who are unable to stand. They must be positioned and radiographed supine, semierect, or seated upright. These films are made generally in anterior-posterior (AP) projection; the position of the patient is supine. However, routine radiographs are made in posterior-anterior (PA) projection; the patient's position is upright. The AP projection tends to magnify anterior structures, such as the heart, and produces a redistribution of blood, thus accentuating upper-lobe vasculature (see Figs. 2–6A and 2–6B). A sharp pleural fluid level that could be visualized in a standard erect film might appear as a diffuse unilateral haziness in the semierect portable roentgenogram (see Chapter 4). Blood vessel and heart size are enhanced in the supine position as demonstrated in Figures 2–6B and 2–6D. Note that the thickest vessels and the largest heart size are seen in an AP supine expiratory film (Fig. 2–6D).

Patient respiration also affects the quality of the image. Chest roentgenography is best done on full inspiration, which allows the greatest amount of lung parenchyma to be visualized. Patients who are short of breath or on ventilatory support may be erroneously radiographed in the expiratory phase of respiration. The heart and the vascular structures are enhanced because of the smaller size of the chest cavity. Figure 2–6 demonstrates positional and respiratory changes in the same person.

EFFECT OF TECHNICAL FACTORS ON IMAGE

Distinguishing a normal radiograph is one of the most important skills of the critical care provider. Normal variations of positions and res-

piration are not the only factors that can significantly alter a chest roentgenogram; technical factors can also have a significant effect on the image.

Overpenetration

Figure 2–7A is a standard PA chest radiograph taken at 90 kV and 1.8 MAS. Notice that the lung is visualized behind the heart, while blood vessels are easily seen permeating the lung parenchyma. Figure 2–7B is a film taken with much higher kV in the same patient. Notice that, while the blood vessels behind the heart are easily seen (*arrow*), the vessels in the lung parenchyma are virtually "burned out," or overpenetrated.

Excessive Milliamperage

The use of excessive milliamperage gives improved tonal qualities and greater anatomic detail. These gains are achieved, however, at much higher radiation levels because increasing milliamperage increases the total number of x-rays produced.

Underpenetration

Figure 2–8A shows an underpenetrated film. Insufficient kilovoltage was used to penetrate the tissues adequately, resulting in low photographic density. Underpenetration produces an inadequate radiograph with lack of anatomic detail because little radiant energy, of varying intensities, is generated that could produce tonal differences on the radiograph. Using higher kilovoltage produces more x-rays of different energies and abilities of tissue penetration, with varying shades on the radiograph. Obesity also may cause relative underpenetration of the film merely on the basis of the increased tissue thickness, (Fig. 2–8B).

Distance

The distance of the subject from the x-ray source affects the image intensity in an inverse fashion. The shorter the source-to-object distance, the more intense is the final image; with greater distance, the radiation and its effects are less intense. Increasing image intensity (density) by using a reduced distance is equivalent to raising milliamperage. It is thus possible to reduce radiation exposure by increasing the subject's distance from the x-ray tube. Chest radiography is usually performed at a distance of six feet, which allows adequate penetration of the low-density lung tissue and minimizes radiation exposure. *(between)*

Distance from the anatomical part and the x-ray film may, in addition, affect image magnification and result in consequent variations in image detail. The farther away the subject is from the cassette (object-to-film distance), the greater is the apparent magnification. The closer the subject is to the film holder, the nearer to actual size is the anatomy represented on the radiograph. For these reasons, the heart appears larger on the AP roentgenogram than on a PA view (see Fig. 2–6). An anterior structure, the heart is positioned farther from the cassette in an AP radiograph when the film is closer to the subject's spine; on a PA film, the cassette is positioned anteriorly—closer to the subject's heart. Thus cardiac magnification is greater in the AP film when the heart is farther from the cassette.

Furthermore, technical errors in positioning can imitate significant intrathoracic diseases. Close scrutiny, however, invariably points to technical errors because the findings are not consistent with the usual roentgenographic patterns of disease. Patient rotation, for example, may mimic an infiltrate, a widened mediastinum, and tracheal deviation (see Fig. 2–9A). The same patient is shown in a near frontal view (Fig. 2–9B); the clavicles are more midpositional (*large arrows*), and the trachea is centered (*small arrows*). Notice how the mediastinum is close to normal width.

Artifacts

An example of film blurring from poor film-screen contact is seen in Figure 2–10 (*arrows*). The lateral clouding is greater on the left than on the right and could mimic several pathologic processes:

- a pleural effusion (However, the costophrenic angle is sharp.)
- an atelectasis (However, the diaphragm is not elevated from loss of volume.)
- an infiltrate (Yet, the lung parenchyma is easily visualized.)

The ultimate answer in discriminating the real from the artifactual is, of course, to repeat the film. If the abnormality suddenly disappears, its artifactual nature is verified.

Figure 2–11 displays several technical problems. Notice the horizontal line of demarcation at the top of the roentgenogram. It is indicative of improper centering of x-ray beam-to-patient-to film. Another technical error that can be seen in Figure 2–11 (which is inexplicable and therefore artifactual) is the opacification and the lucency shown laterally. The *arrows* point to increased density that passes out of the lung fields into the axilla. Pulmonary parenchymal disease is not likely to cause this. The same holds true for the increased lucency (shown at the arrowhead tips) that passes from lung parenchyma to the axilla. This condition is not subcutaneous emphysema because the lucency crosses the rib; it does not follow the contour, as it often does in the case of subcutaneous air. Furthermore, this artifactual lucency is less well-defined than is subcutaneous air.

Other extraneous artifacts seen in the critical care arena may make roentgenographic interpretation confusing and difficult. Figure 2–12 shows cardiac monitoring leads (*large arrow*). The radiopaque tip of the nasogastric tube is observed outside the patient (*white arrow*). Figure 2–13 shows the radiopaque bars of a Stryker frame used by a cervical fracture patient with bilateral aspiration pneumonia.

RADIATION BIOLOGY

X-rays have the capability of damaging living tissue in proportion to the level of exposure over a given period. This damage can be in the form of genetic or somatic abnormalities. Chromosomal damage and mutation are among some of the genetic aberrations produced. Somatic damage includes skin damage, radiation pneumonitis, radiation sickness, and death.

The amount of radiation to patients undergoing chest roentgenography is relatively small when compared to other radiographic examinations and is relatively benign when the exposure that would be necessary to cause tissue damage is considered. For example, a portable chest x-ray examination results in about 44 mR of skin exposure; whereas a barium enema would yield approximately 1,320 mR of skin exposure. Considering that the maximum permissible dose of radiation to the general population per year is 500 mR, the average adult would have to receive 11 chest examinations to exceed this limit.

Hospital personnel should always be concerned about levels of radiation exposure during roentgenography in the intensive care unit. Herman states that the average exposure for nonoccupational workers in a four-bed intensive care unit was 0.05 mR a week. This translates to an exposure of 2.6 mR per year—well below the 500 mR limit imposed by the National Council on Radiation Protection for the general population.

REFERENCES

Herman W, Patrick J, Tabrisky J: A comparative study of scattered radiation levels from 80-KUP and 240-KUP x-rays in the surgical intensive care unit. *Radiology* 1980; 137:552–553.

Johns KE, Cunningham JR: *Physics of Radiology,* ed 3. Springfield, Ill, Charles C Thomas Publishers, 1971, pp 639, 642.

Solman J: *The Fundamentals of X-ray and Radium Physics,* ed 6. Springfield, Ill, Charles C Thomas Publishers, 1978, pp 515, 530–532.

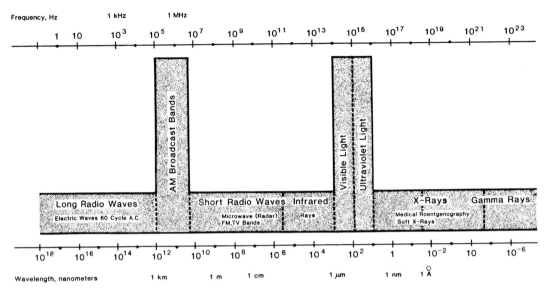

Figure 2–1. Electromagnetic spectrum. Notice that x-rays are in the shorter wavelength, higher frequency area.

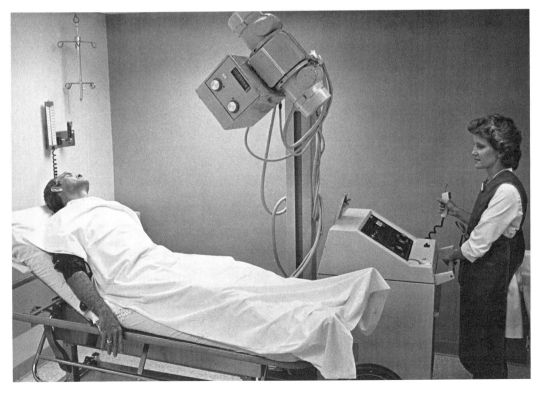

Figure 2–2. Positioning patient for mobile chest radiograph. Cassette is located posteriorly between patient and bed.

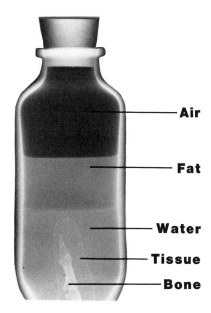

Figure 2–3. Glass container. Radiograph compares various densities of the human body.

— Air

— Fat

— Water

— Tissue

— Bone

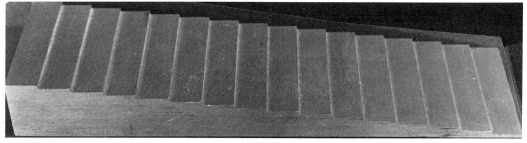

Level a   Level b

Figure 2–4A. Step wedge for checking radiographic techniques. **A.** Metal step wedge.

Level a   Level b

Figure 2–4B. Radiograph demonstrates the variance of x–ray exposure with thickness of wedge.

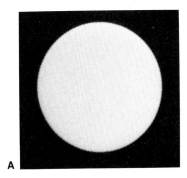 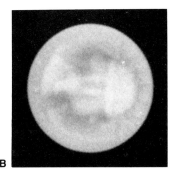

A   **B**

Figure 2–5. Scale of contrast. **A.** Radiograph of a coin at low kV demonstrating short scale of contrast. **B.** At high kV, displaying long scale contrast.

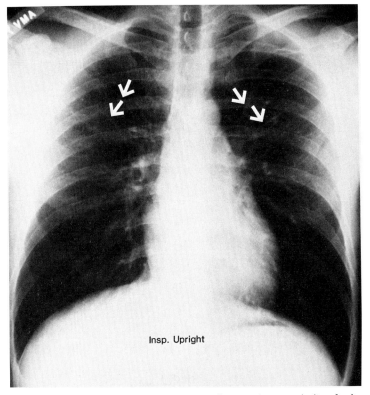

Insp. Upright

Figure 2–6A. Positional and respiratory changes in vascularity. **A.** An inspiratory PA upright chest film. Note sparse upper lobe vasculature caused by normal gravitational effects (*white arrows*).

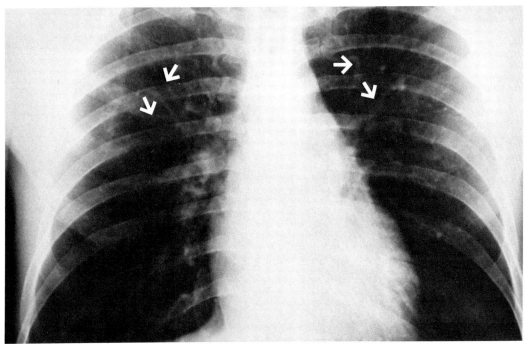

Figure 2–6B. An inspiratory AP supine film. Note in the same patient the hyperemia and the thicker vessels (*white arrows*), secondary to gravitational changes; also the larger heart size than that seen in PA film—also due to gravitational effects in addition to magnification.

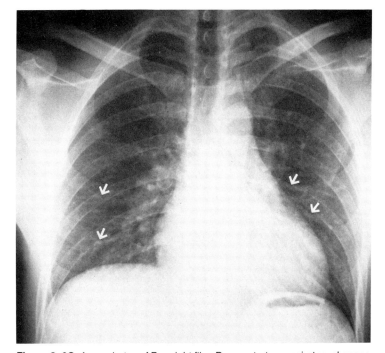

Figure 2–6C. An expiratory AP upright film. Demonstrates respiratory changes in vascularity of patient when expiration is during upright position; arrows point to enhanced lower lobe vasculature when compared to Figure A or Figure B.

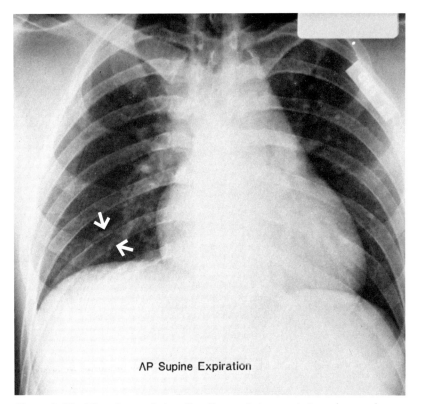

AP Supine Expiration

Figure 2–6D. AP supine expiratory film. Demonstrates respiratory changes in vascularity when patient is supine. Expiration causes reduction in thoracic cage volume and relative shortening and thickening of vascular structures (*white arrows*).

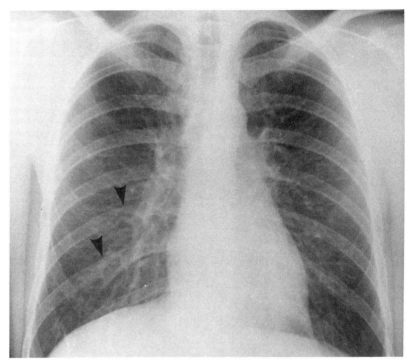

Figure 2–7A. Alterations in appearances on chest radiographs using high and low kV techniques. Low kV.

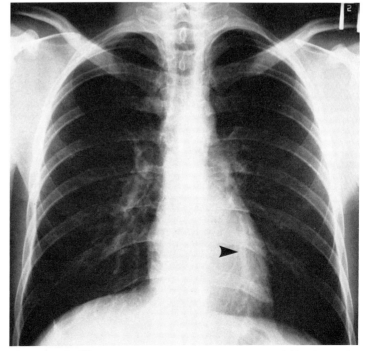

Figure 2–7B. High kV. Note differences in sharpness of blood vessels (*arrows*) with changes in kV.

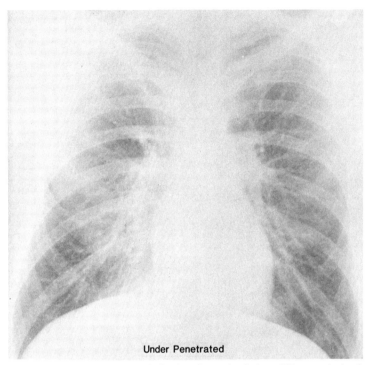

Figure 2–8A. Underpenetrated chest radiograph. **A.** Low kV—note lack of diagnostic detail.

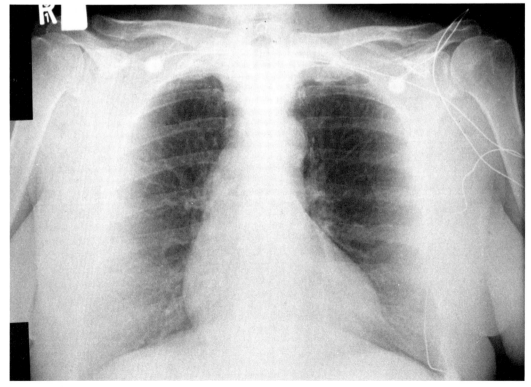

Figure 2–8B. In an obese patient.

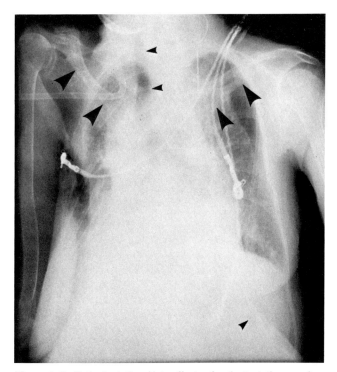

Figure 2–9. Patient rotation. Note effects of patient rotation on mimicking a pathologic process. **A.** Patient is rotated.

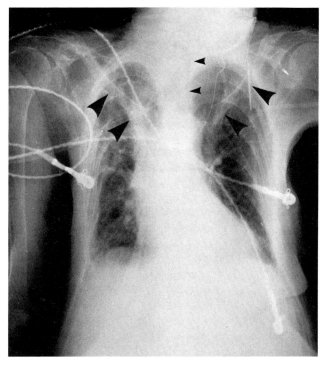

Figure 2–9B. Position is more nearly normal. Note rotation of clavicles (*large arrows*); *small arrows* show changes in position of trachea.

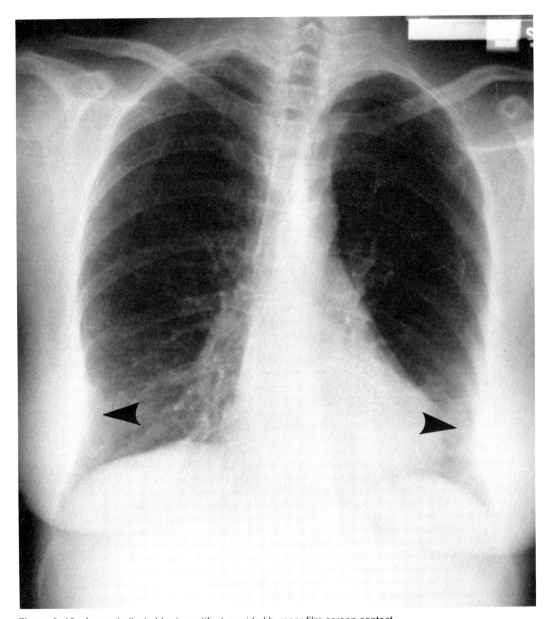

Figure 2–10. *Arrows* indicate blurring artifact provided by poor film-screen contact.

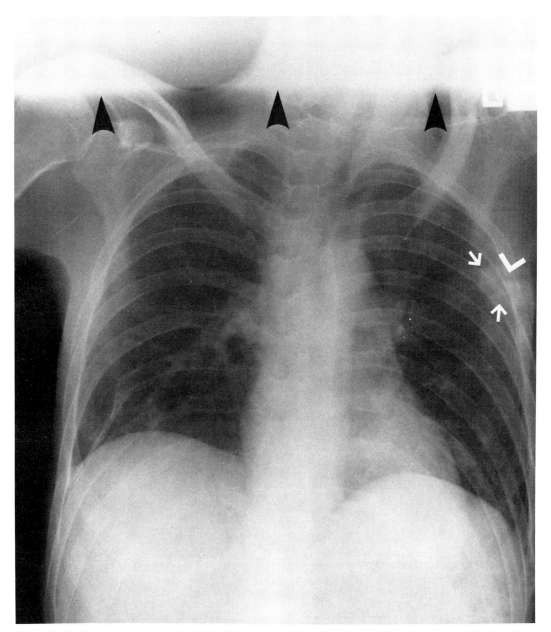

Figure 2–11. Examples of technical artifacts; *black arrows* delineate beam cutoff from improper positioning of the patient in relation to x-ray beam. The *white arrows* and *arrowhead* represent pressure artifacts.

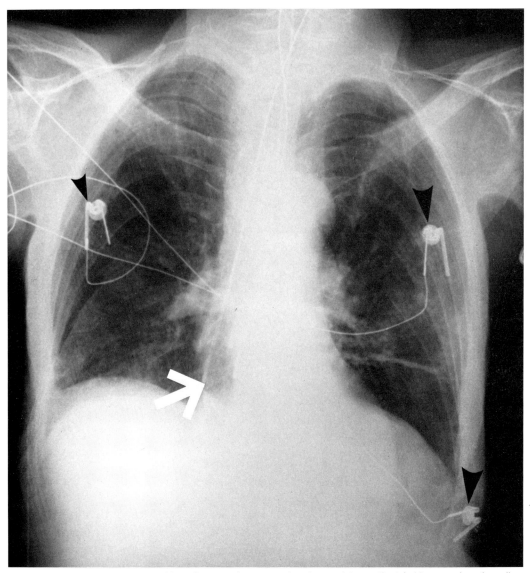

Figure 2–12. Artifacts are provided here by part of nasogastric tube overlying patient (*white arrow*) and cardiac monitoring electrodes (*black arrows*).

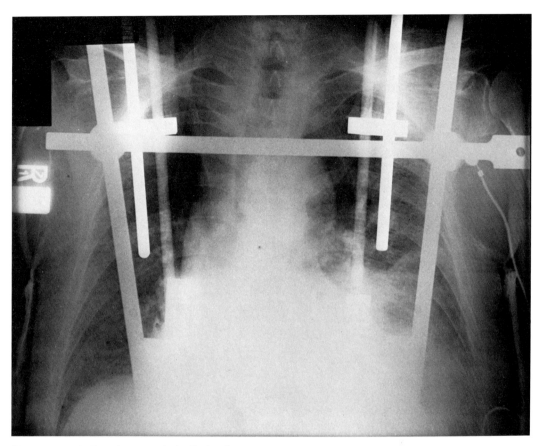

Figure 2–13. Artifacts from metal of a Stryker frame.

Chapter 3

Abnormal Roentgenographic Patterns

Lyle D. Victor, MD, *James I. Breckenfeld*, MD, *and Allen J. Stone*, MD

Diseased lung tissues have easily recognizable patterns that can be divided into localized and diffuse processes. These geographic divisions can be further divided into more anatomically discrete pathophysiologic descriptions: alveolar, interstitial, reticular, nodular, and bronchial disease patterns.

LOCALIZED DISEASE PROCESSES

Infiltrates are localized roentgenographic processes involving the abnormal movement of substances into alveolar or interstitial (lung connective tissue) spaces. They frequently follow a lobar or segmental distribution.

A typical example of localized infiltrative disease is the pneumonic process seen in Figure 3–1, which shows a left lower lobe pneumonia. Notice the whitish area at the left lung base (*asterisk*). The dome of the left hemidiaphragm is poorly visualized (*arrowheads*) because the infiltrate increases the density of the involved lung, which is normally filled with air.

As its weight per unit volume (density) approaches that of soft tissue, the line of demarcation between diaphragm and lung becomes obscured and creates the *silhouette* sign. Notice the preservation of the left margin of the heart; it indicates the posterior location of the infiltrate. Another left lower lobe pneumonia that involves the most apical portion of the lobe is the superior segment infiltrate seen in Figures 3–2A and

3–2B. The lateral view demonstrates the posterior location of the segment filled with infiltrate. Aspiration pneumonia frequently involves this area because the superior segment bronchus takes off posteriorly, which makes this segment gravity dependent in a supine patient. This body placement is the most frequently encountered in the debilitated, hospitalized patient.

A right lower lobe infiltrate is demonstrated in Figure 3–3A. The infiltrate results in a silhouette sign at the right side of the diaphragm. Because the border of the heart is easily seen, the possibility of right middle lobe involvement (*arrows*) is reduced. An infiltrate in the middle lobe usually obliterates the anterior right margin of the heart. The lateral view provides further useful anatomic delineation. The *arrows* in Figure 3–3B outline the normal course of the major fissure that obliquely crosses the lung field. The increased inferior density (*asterisk*) marks the total infiltration or consolidation of the right lower lobe. Although lateral views are very useful in clarifying the anatomic relationships seen on the PA film, they are not routinely done in the intensive care unit because the portable units are not powerful enough to get adequate posterior penetration of tissue, which is required by the increased tissue thickness when shooting x-ray films in this position.

Infiltrates in the various segments of the right middle lobe are seen in Figures 3–4 and 3–5. Figure 3–4A shows visual loss of the right border of the heart, which signifies involvement of the medial segment. The diaphragm is completely visualized, which verifies that the right lower lobe is not involved because the right middle lobe does not anatomically abut the diaphragm. The lateral view seen in Figure 3–4B shows a typical anterior and midlung field location (*asterisk*). Involvement of the lateral segment of the right middle lobe is shown in Figure 3–5A. There is no silhouetting of either the right border of the heart or the right side of the diaphragm. Figure 3–5 demonstrates the consolidation marginated by the minor fissure above (*large dark arrow*) and by the major fissure below (*small open arrows*).

Klebsiella pneumonia may appear as an expansile consolidative process (Fig. 3–6). The *arrows* point to the minor fissure, which is depressed downward by the enlarging infiltrate. The *asterisk* denotes a consolidative process. If a pathologic process diffusely involves a whole lobe or segment, it can be said to be consolidated. The physical findings of bronchial breathing and dullness to percussion are often noted. Bronchial breath sounds are higher pitched breath sounds and are clearly heard because sound travels better through denser material. (Remember hearing boat motors better from far away when your head was submerged at the lake last summer?) The diffuse ''ground glass'' appearance of this infiltrate, sometimes called an alveolar process, represents alveolar filling at a microscopic level. There are many pathophysiologic processes that can cause an alveolar process—from the diffuse alveolar filling in pulmonary edema to the inflammatory exudate seen in pneumonitis. An alveolar process can be manifested by alveoli filled with blood, exudate, protein, or neoplasm.

Aspiration pneumonia can be localized and diffuse (Fig. 3–7). The localized form is seen in the x-ray film of a child who swallowed kerosene and developed subsequent hydrocarbon aspiration pneumonitis (Figs. 3–7A and 3–7B). The *shaded arrow* points to the left lower lobe infiltrate. The *open* and *closed arrows* denote the less dense kerosene floating in the top of the fluid-filled stomach.

LOCALIZED LUNG DISEASE

Atelectasis

Abnormal loss of lung volume is known as atelectasis or collapse. Because small amounts of atelectasis can be associated with increasing shunt fractions and hypoxemia (resulting in dramatic deterioration of a patient's clinical status), a thorough understanding of the roentgenographic presentations of atelectasis is necessary.

Figures 3–8A, 3–8B, and 3–8C show sequential development of atelectasis of the right lower lobe in a patient with a malfunctioning right hemidiaphragm. Figure 3–8A is an unremarkable film taken immediately after surgery for a perforated peptic ulcer. A film made 12 hours later (Fig. 3–8B) demonstrates subsegmental atelectasis manifested by horizontal, streaking densities (*large arrows*); the right hemidiaphragm could not descend normally to allow optimal expansion of the lung. More advanced atelectasis with loss of volume of the right lower lobe and the middle lobe is seen in Figure 3–8C.

Total collapse of the left upper lobe from a mucus plug is seen in Figure 3–9A. The primarily upper–lobe nature of this process is suggested by the intact left margin of the diaphragm (*arrowheads*). The main clue to upper–lobe involvement is the loss of the silhouette of the left margin of the heart. Figure 3–9B is a film of the same patient after adequate suctioning.

Figure 3–10A shows total collapse of the left lung from pooled secretions in an emphysema patient with chronic aspiration. There is now a silhouette sign of the left margin of the heart and the left hemidiaphragm margin. After fiberoptic bronchoscopy was performed, the left upper lobe re–expanded (Fig. 3–10B). The remaining obliteration of the left hemidiaphragm margin and the margin of the heart indicated continued consolidation of the lingula and the left lower lobe. Figure 3–10C shows the left lung fully expanded after postural drainage, chest physical therapy, and bronchodilator therapy. Notice the typical hyperexpansion of the lungs and the flattening of the diaphragm often seen in chronic obstructive pulmonary disease (COPD) patients (see also Fig. 3–34).

Figure 3–11 shows atelectasis of the right middle and lower lobes, secondary to a tumor mass. Lung cancer patients often develop atelectasis because the increasing mass causes bronchial obstruction resulting in respiratory insufficiency, which requires ventilatory support. Notice the tracheal deviation to the right, partly from patient rotation but mostly from loss of volume and compensatory hyperexpansion of the left lung. Lung hyperexpansion is suspected on the left because of the paucity of blood vessels and the fullness of the lung fields when compared with the right lung. Complete collapse secondary to a tumor is seen in Figure 3–12. The *large arrow* points to the "cut–off" right mainstem bronchus, which is totally occluded with tumor. The left main and upper lobe bronchi are compressed by a tumor mass (*small arrows*).

Neoplasms

Lung cancer has many localized roentgenographic manifestations. The patient with alveolar cell carcinoma (Fig. 3–13A) had an infiltrate in the lingula. Figure 3–13B is a tomogram showing an air bronchogram, which is a normal air-filled bronchus surrounded by a lung with increased density. The alveolar cell carcinoma or bronchoalveolar cell carcinoma consists of neoplastic epithelial cells lining the alveoli and creating the appearance of an alveolar infiltrate. The bronchial structure is left intact, however, and thus creates the air bronchograms often seen in this disorder.

The patient whose chest film is shown in Figure 3–14 was admitted to the critical care unit complaining of severe right shoulder pain. The apical opacification suggested in Figure 3–14A is more apparent in the shoulder views in Figure 3–14B (*asterisk*). Figure 3–14C shows the typical rib destruction associated with a Pancoast's or superior sulcus tumor (*arrows*).

Figure 3–15A shows a mass superimposed over the right hilum. Its sharp interface with the

lung suggests that this is a mediastinal mass pushing the mediastinal pleura in a lateral direction (*arrows*). The mass was a thymoma located in the anterior mediastinal space of the anterior chest. It can be seen on the lateral view, Figure 3–15B (*arrows*).

Figure 3–16 shows an example of metastatic cancer. Each *asterisk* marks a "cannon-ball" lesion in this patient with malignant melanoma.

Radiation pneumonitis can result from radiation therapy to the chest for a malignant neoplasm. Inflammation from radiation is usually easy to distinguish because it closely follows radiation ports as shown in Figure 3–17 (*arrows*). This woman had a right perihilar bronchogenic carcinoma with mediastinal involvement and 3,500 rads of radiation therapy to the mediastinum and right anterior chest. Three months later, she developed acute dyspnea and hypoxemia, which required mechanical ventilation and steroid therapy.

Cavities

Carcinoma of the lung can cavitate or can obstruct a bronchus with subsequent infectious cavitation or abscess formation. An example of an abscess in a patient with an obstructed superior segment from a squamous cell carcinoma is shown in Figures 3–18A and 3–18B. The *arrows* mark the air-fluid level contained in the cavity. Copious, purulent, foul smelling pus was removed at bronchoscopy, leaving only residual infiltrates (Fig. 3–18C).

Septic pulmonary emboli can form multiple lung parenchymal cavities like those shown in Figure 3–19A (*arrows*). The lateral view (Fig. 3–19B) shows a good example of the thickened, inflamed outer wall. The source of the infected material was septic thrombophlebitis.

Tuberculosis commonly causes tissue destruction and cavity formation (Fig. 3–20). Reactivation tuberculosis most commonly involves the apical segments of the upper lobes (*arrows*). A miliary pattern is occasionally seen; it is described below.

A pneumatocele is a cystic space that may develop in young patients who have staphylococcal pneumonia. They often have fluid levels like that seen in Figures 3–21A and 3–21B. They resolve spontaneously after several weeks.

Bronchiectasis is the breakdown of bronchial structure secondary to inflammation. Prominent linear streaks representing the damaged bronchial wall may be seen. Occasionally ring shadows are found. They represent a dilated, inflamed bronchus seen end-on—Figure 3–22 (*white arrow*).

DIFFUSE LUNG DISEASE

Aspiration Syndromes

Aspiration pneumonia can appear as a localized and a diffuse process. Figure 3–23A is an x-ray film of a patient with multiple sclerosis who had dysphagia and recurrent aspiration of pharyngeal contents. This disorder is marked by primarily lower-lobe infiltrates because, in the case of the upright patient, gravity propels aspirated material to the dependent lower lobes. Figure 3–23B is an esophagram of the same patient. The *large white arrows* point to barium in the pharynx. The *smaller white arrows* point to aspirated barium in the tracheobronchial tree on the right. The *black arrows* point to barium in the esophagus.

The upper lobes also can be involved in aspiration syndromes because the posterior segment of the right upper lobe and the apical-posterior segment of the left upper lobe exit the upper lobe bronchi posteriorly and are in a dependent position when the patient lies on his back. Aspirated contents can then flow dorsally with the aid of gravitation, which occurred in the patient shown in Figure 3–24—just before the induction of anesthesia. The *asterisks* mark the predominantly involved upper lobes.

Other infections can cause diffuse lung diseases often seen in the critical care unit. Miliary tuberculosis appears as multiple uniformly sized nodules, so called because of their size and similarity to millet seeds (Fig. 3–25).

Adult Respiratory Distress Syndrome

The adult respiratory distress syndrome (ARDS), sometimes called shock lung, appears as diffuse alveolar infiltrates. Some of the multiple etiologies of this disorder include infection, sepsis, shock, pancreatitis, and toxic fume inhalation. Figure 3–26 shows a series of roentgenograms of a patient with ARDS as a result of pneumococcal pneumonia; she could not be weaned from intubation and positive end expiratory pressure because of persistent hypoxemia.

The x-ray film shown in Figure 3–26A is a film taken just after intubation. Ventilation and positive end expiratory pressure (PEEP) were initiated, which resulted in improved aeration (Fig. 3–26B). PEEP increases the functional residual capacity and thereby increases the total amount of gas in the lung after end-tidal respiration on the ventilator. This increase accounts for the appearance of decreased fluid in the lung fields when, in fact, the lungs have improved expansion. A roentgenogram taken a few days later showed an almost normal lung (Fig. 3–26C). The patient's vital capacity, minute ventilation, and maximum inspiratory force were all normal. She was rapidly weaned from ventilatory support and PEEP and was extubated. Six hours later, she required reintubation because of tachypnea and hypoxia. Figure 3–26D shows the "recurrent" pulmonary edema.

The diffuse alveolar damage that occurs in cases of the ARDS may take up to three weeks, or more, to heal. Weaning from mechanical ventilation may be possible, but continued PEEP is often necessary to maintain alveolar patency and adequate oxygenation. The "recurrent" pulmonary edema is not really recurrent; it is actually the appearance of increased density previously masked by the increased volume of gas in the lung made possible by PEEP.

Miscellaneous Diffuse Processes

Toxic disease processes frequently involve the alveolar and bronchiolar anatomy in a diffuse fashion. The roentgenogram shown in Figure

3–27A is that of a young man who inhaled chlorine gas. He subsequently developed shortness of breath and severe hypoxemia. A diffuse alveolar nodular pattern is present and is more apparent on the right than on the left (*arrows*). Figure 3–27B is a normal roentgenogram of the same patient two weeks later.

Uremic patients (Fig. 3–28) may be in respiratory distress with diffuse alveolar infiltrates. The exact etiology of this process in renal failure is unknown.

Lymphagitic spread of carcinoma may appear as a diffuse interstitial process. Figure 3–29 is a film of a 60-year-old man with metastatic adenocarcinoma. The *large arrowheads* point to Kerley's A lines, which represent carcinomatous infiltration of the perihilar lymphatics. The meniscus of a pleural effusion is marked by an *asterisk*.

Respiratory insufficiency secondary to vasculitis may appear as a diffuse parenchymal process in a patient with Wegener's granulomatosis (Fig. 3–30). Enough tissue destruction can occur to cause cavities (*arrowheads*). Acute respiratory failure with diffuse infiltrates also can be seen in patients with disorders of uncertain etiology. The patient in Figure 3–31 came with a typical presentation of Goodpasture's syndrome: hematuria, uremia, hemoptysis, and progressive anemia. Goodpasture's syndrome was confirmed by renal biopsy, which showed an acute glomerular nephritis. The pulmonary infiltrates may be secondary to intraalveolar hemorrhage, the exact etiology of which is unclear.

Diffuse infiltrations of the lungs by inorganic material, followed by subsequent development of interstitial fibrosis, can occur in occupational lung diseases. Figure 3–32 is a roentgenogram of a patient with simple silicosis. Note the diffuse interstitial nodularity throughout the lungs. The nodules are well-demarcated, which is characteristic of the interstitial location. The *arrows* in Figure 3–33 demonstrate a mass in the right upper lobe whose margins parallel the lateral chest margin. This condition is the hallmark of progressive massive fibrosis—the complicated form of silicosis.

Diffuse lung disease can also show decreased density like that seen in a patient with severe emphysema (Figs. 3–34A and 3–34B). The darker appearance of the hyperlucent, hyperexpanded lung fields is a typical finding when there has been extensive loss of alveolar structure and lung elasticity and an increase in air trapping. A relative lack of vascularity and a flattening of the hemidiaphragms are also frequent findings. The lateral view verifies the flattened diaphragm in this patient with congenital α_1-antitrypsin deficiency. Acute bronchospasm can increase air trapping and thus enhance all the findings cited above. The retrosternal air space may also be increased in some patients; however, in the above roentgenogram, it was normal.

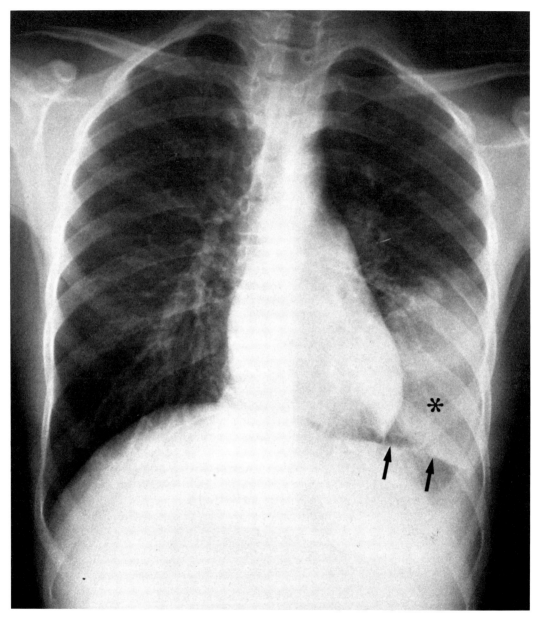

Figure 3–1. Left lower lobe pneumonitis (*asterisk*). Note partial obscuration of left hemidiaphragm (*arrows*) and preservation of left border of the heart.

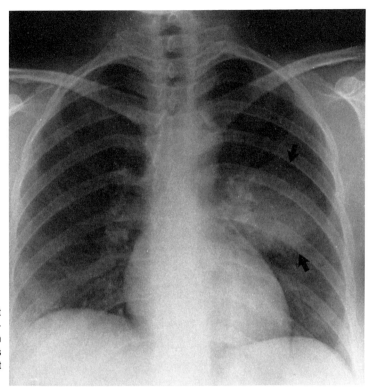

Figure 3–2. Superior segment infiltrate. **A.** Left mid lung consolidation (*arrows*) with preservation of left margin of the heart suggests involvement of superior segment of left lower lobe.

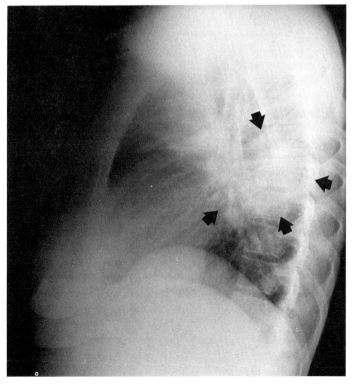

Figure 3–2B. Lateral view confirms posterior location of infiltrate in superior segment of left lower lobe (*arrows*).

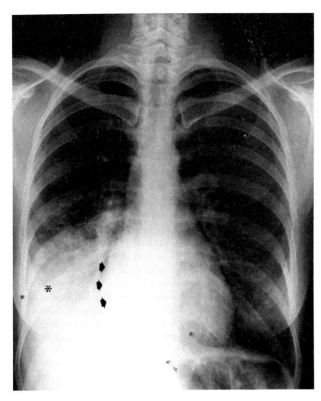

Figure 3–3A. Right lower lobe infiltrate. Consolidation (*asterisk*) demonstrates loss of silhouette with hemidiaphragm; note preservation of right margin of the heart (*arrows*), indicating no involvement of the more anterior middle lobe.

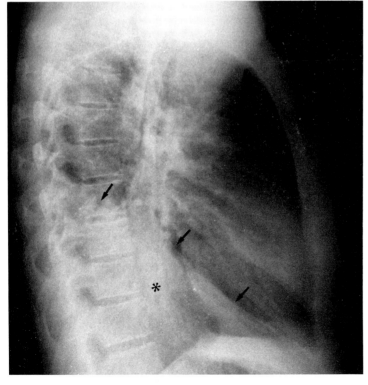

Figure 3–3B. Lateral view demonstrates major or oblique fissure (*arrows*) well-delineated by right lower lobe consolidation (*asterisk*) and anterior aerated right upper lobe and right middle lobe.

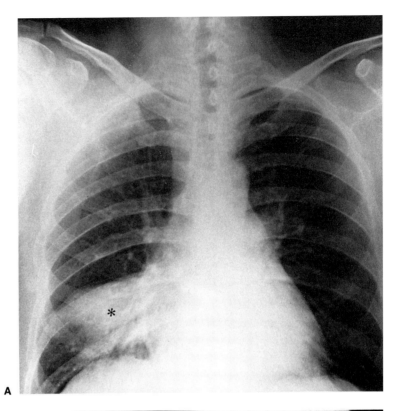

A

Figure 3–4. Infiltrates of medial segment of right middle lobe. **A.** Note consolidation of right middle lobe (*asterisk*); note also obscuration of right margin of the heart, indicating involvement of the medial segment. **B.** Lateral view displays the anterior consolidation of the middle lobe (*asterisk*).

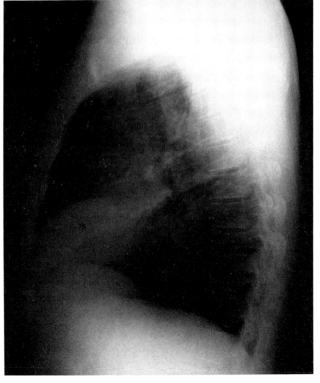

B

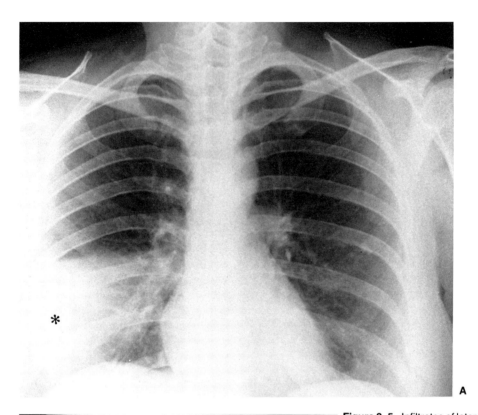

A

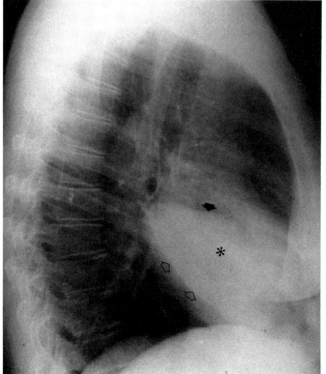

Figure 3–5. Infiltrates of lateral segment of right middle lobe. **A.** Note that consolidation of the lateral segment of the middle lobe (*asterisk*) does not affect right margin of the heart or right hemidiaphragm. **B.** Lateral view demonstrates consolidation of the middle lobe (*asterisk*) between the minor fissure (*black arrow*) and the major fissure (*open arrows*).

B

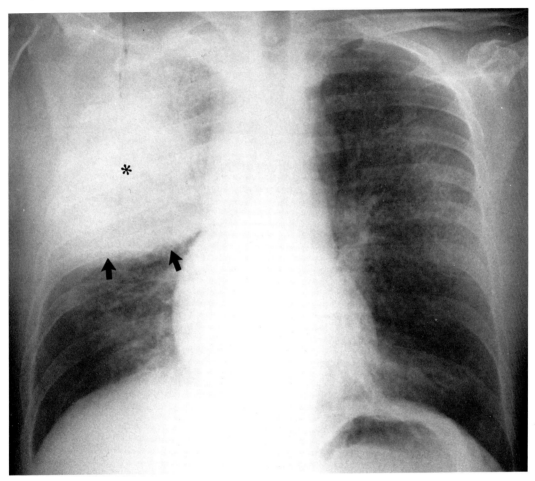

Figure 3–6. Patient with Klebsiella pneumonia. Note expansile consolidation of the right upper lobe (*asterisk*), causing downward depression of the minor fissure (*arrows*).

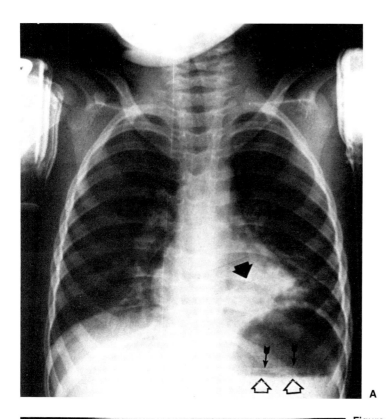

A

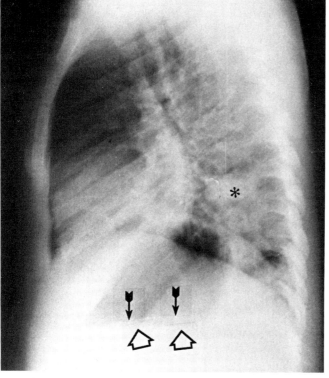

B

Figure 3–7. Localized aspiration pneumonia. **A.** Aspiration pneumonitis of left lower lobe (*shaded arrow*) is due to aspiration of kerosene. Note air-fluid level in the stomach (*open arrows*); a second level above this level is due to less dense kerosene (*small arrows*). **B.** The lateral view confirms posterior location of infiltrate (*asterisk*).

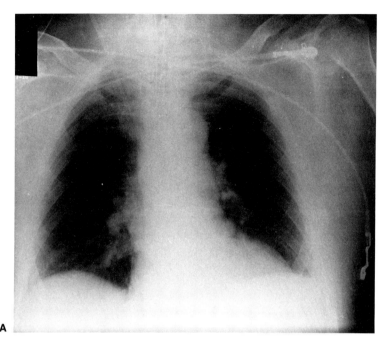

A

Figure 3–8. Sequential development of atelectasis. **A.** Portable chest x-ray film after abdominal surgery shows no active identifiable process. **B.** 12 hours later, subsegmental postoperative atelectasis developed at right lung base (*large arrows*); note margins of right hemidiaphragm (*small arrows*).

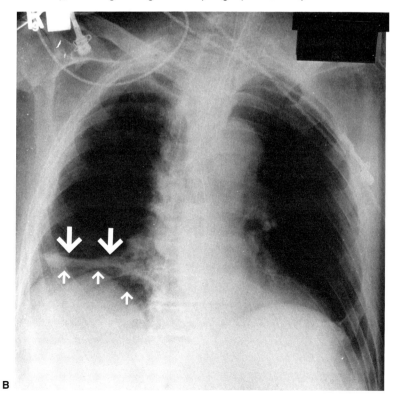

B

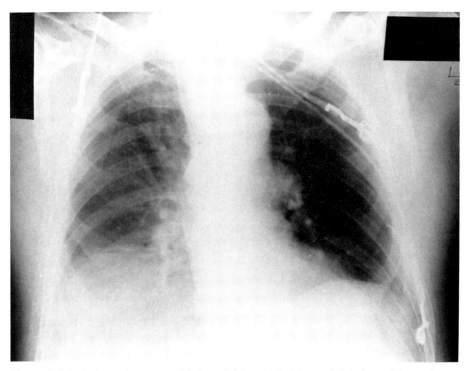

Figure 3–8C. 24 hours later, consolidation of right middle lobe and right lower lobe is due to atelectasis; loss of right hemidiaphragm margin and right margin of the heart is due to silhouette sign.

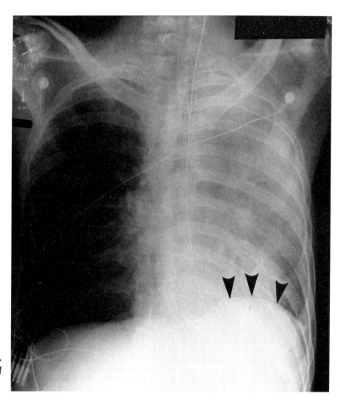

Figure 3–9. Left upper lobe atelectasis. **A.** Note elevation of the preserved margin of the left hemidiaphragm (*arrowheads*).

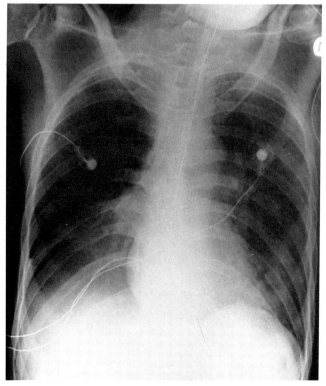

Figure 3–9B. Marked improvement is shown after suctioning.

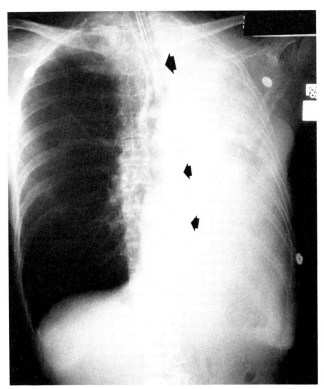

Figure 3–10. Emphysema patient with chronic aspiration. **A.** Total collapse of left lung results in shift of trachea (*large arrow*) and NG tube in esophagus (*small arrows*) to the left because of volume loss.

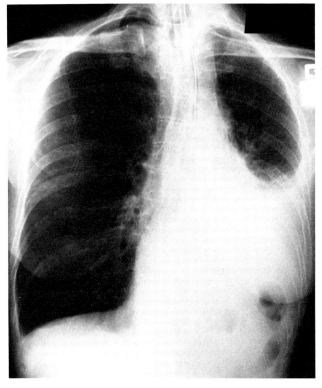

Figure 3–10B. After suctioning, there is partial aeration of left upper lobe and residual atelectasis of lingula characterized by obliteration of left margin of the heart. Obliteration of left hemidiaphragm indicates atelectasis of left lower lobe.

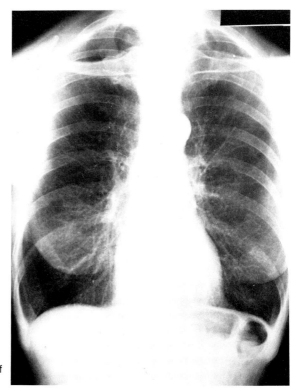

Figure 3–10C. Subsequent total clearing of atelectasis has taken place.

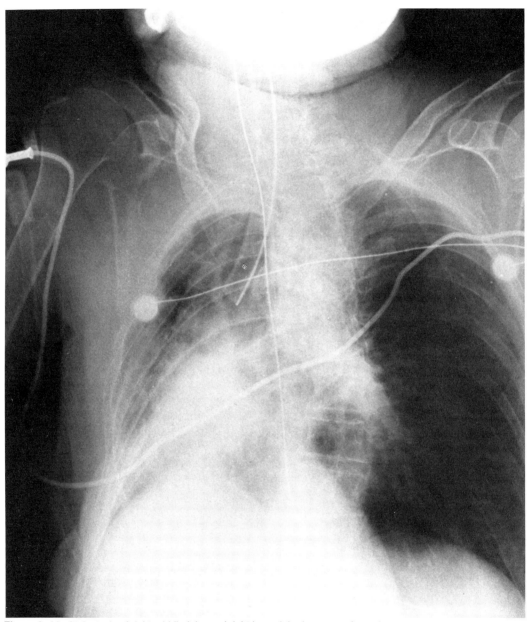

Figure 3–11. Atelectasis of right middle lobe and right lower lobe because of neoplasm.

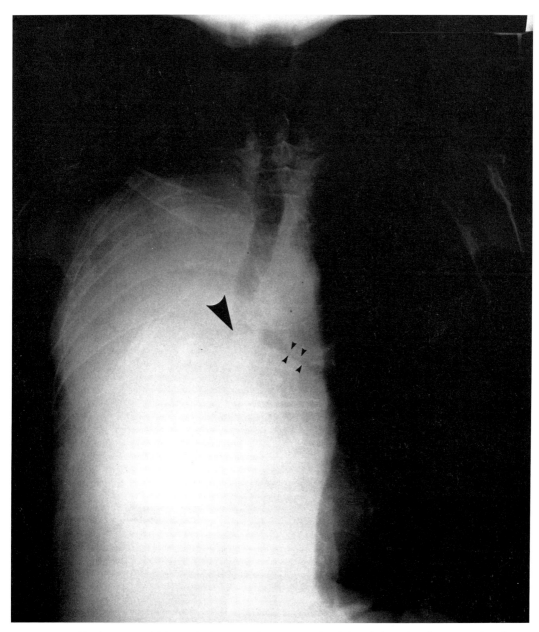

Figure 3–12. Total collapse of right lung is due to neoplasm obstructing right main bronchus (*large arrowhead*); note also severely narrowed left main and upper lobe bronchi (*small arrowheads*), which is due to neoplasm.

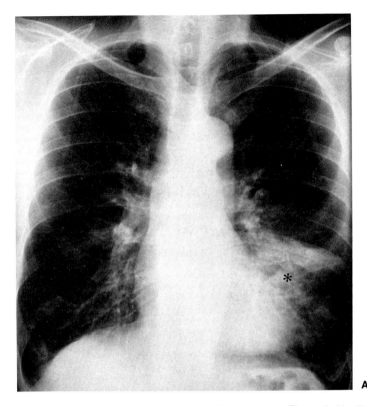

A

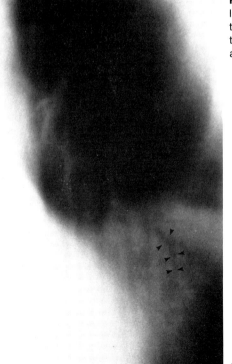

Figure 3–13. Alveolar cell carcinoma. **A.** Appears as lingular infiltrate (*asterisk*); note the loss of left border of the heart. **B.** Laminography demonstrates characteristic air bronchograms seen with this neoplasm. Note air filled bronchus surrounded by neoplasm (*arrows*).

B

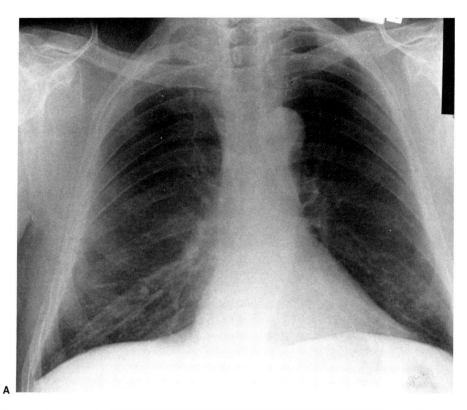

A

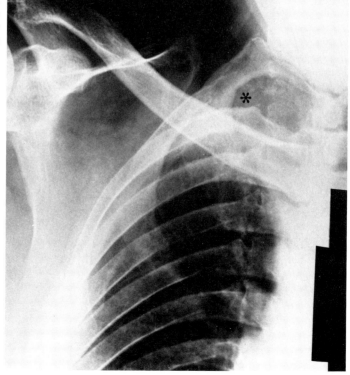

B

Figure 3–14. Pancoast's tumor. **A.** Apical opacification on right is due to neoplasm. **B.** Right shoulder x-ray film demonstrates opacification (*asterisk*).

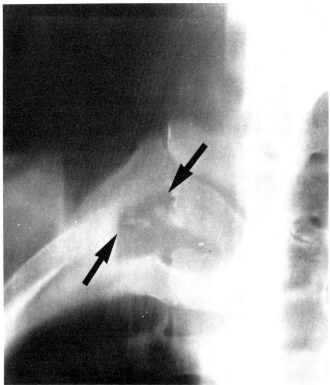

Figure 3–14C. Tomography displays rib destruction (*arrows*) due to neoplasm.

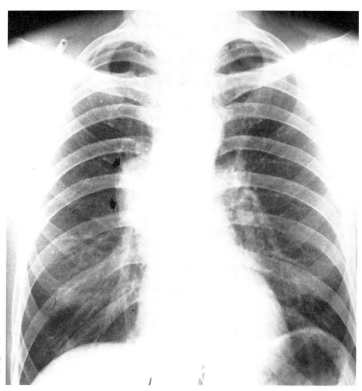

Figure 3–15. Mediastinal mass. **A.** Smooth-margined mass is superimposed over the right hilum (*arrows*).

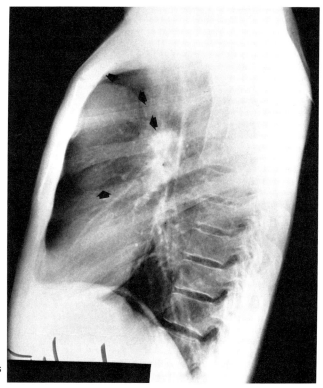

B. Lateral view displays anterior mass (*arrows*) representing a thymoma.

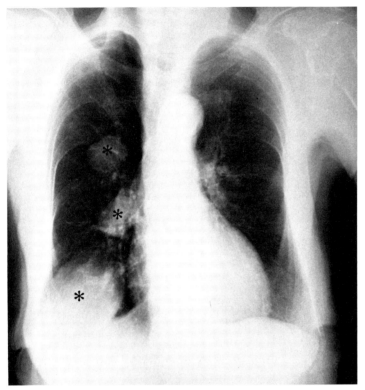

Figure 3–16. Multiple metastatic masses (*asterisks*).

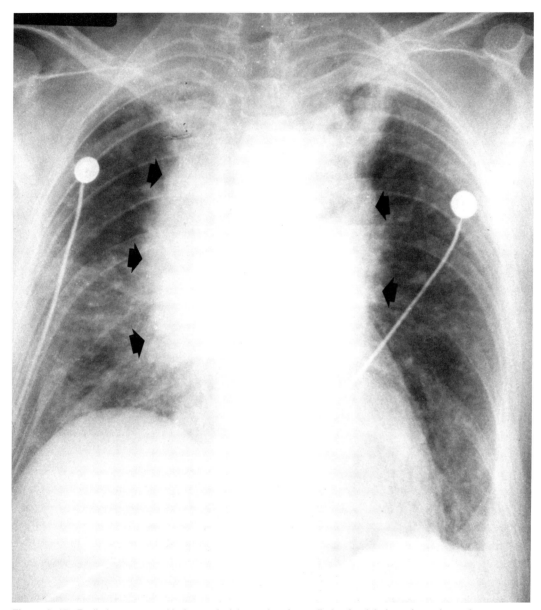

Figure 3–17. Radiation pneumonitis (*arrows*) eight weeks after radiation for right bronchogenic carcinoma.

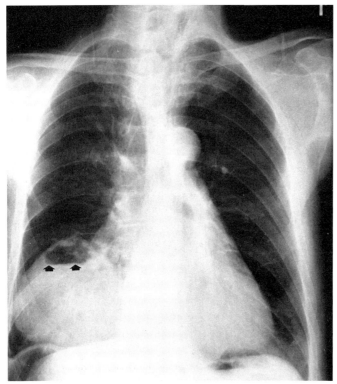

Figure 3–18. Abscess right lower lobe.
A. Note air-fluid level of abscess (*arrows*).

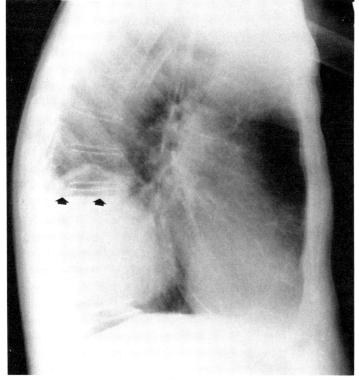

Figure 3–18B. Lateral view demonstrates posterior location of abscess in lower lobe.

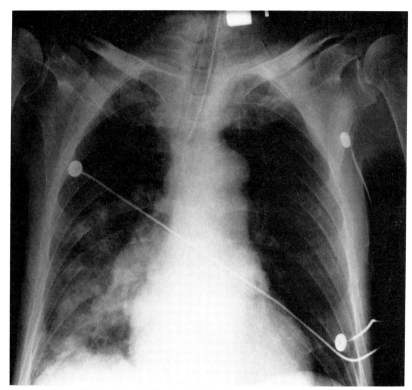

Figure 3–18C. Note residual infiltrate after bronchoscopic aspiration of abscess.

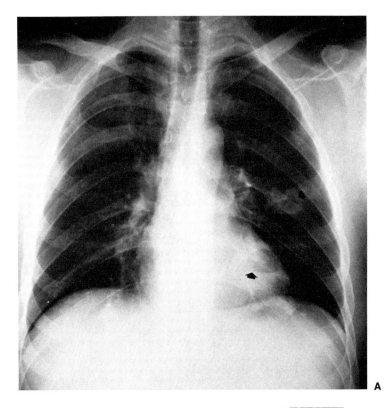

A

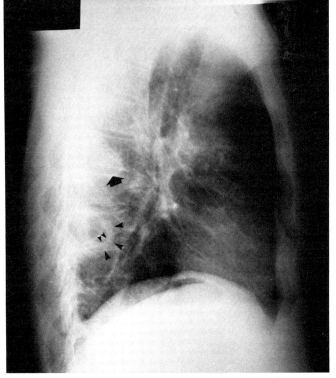

B

Figure 3–19. Lung parenchymal cavities. **A.** Septic emboli causing cavities (*arrows*). **B.** Lateral view demonstrates thickened cavity walls (*arrowheads*). The *arrow* points to superiorly located cavity.

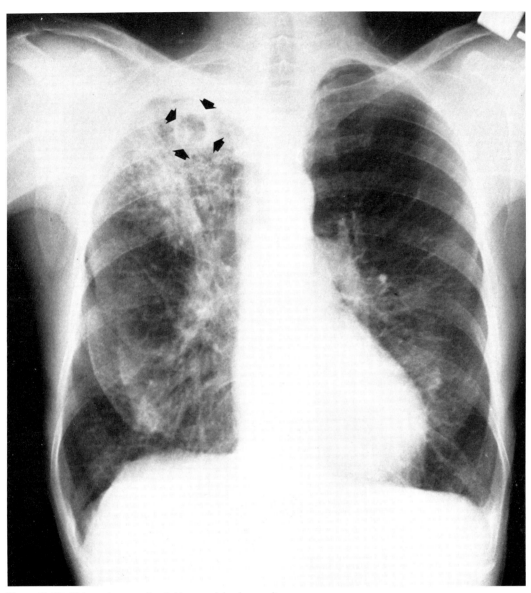

Figure 3–20. Tuberculous cavity, right upper lobe (*arrows*).

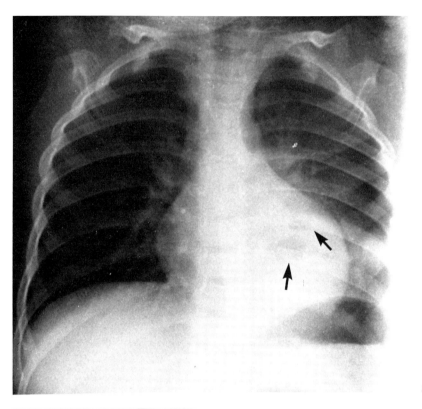

A

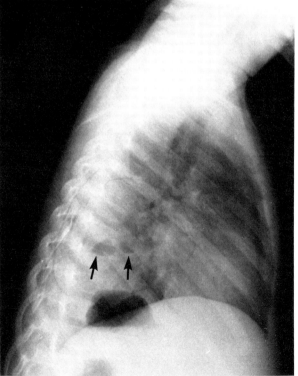

B

Figure 3–21. Cystic space. **A.** Pneumatocele in child recovering from staphylococcal pneumonia (*arrows*). **B.** Lateral view demonstrates air-fluid level (*arrows*).

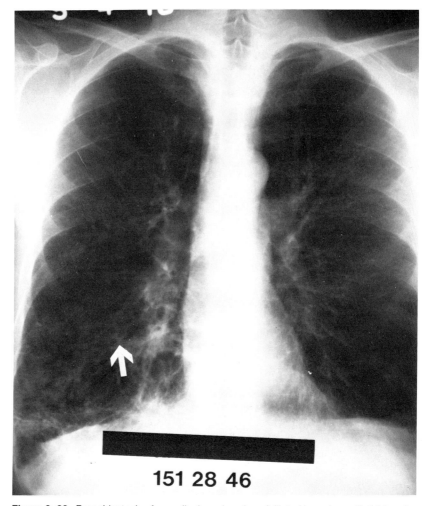

151 28 46

Figure 3–22. Bronchiectasis. *Arrow* displays ring sign of dilated bronchus with thick wall.

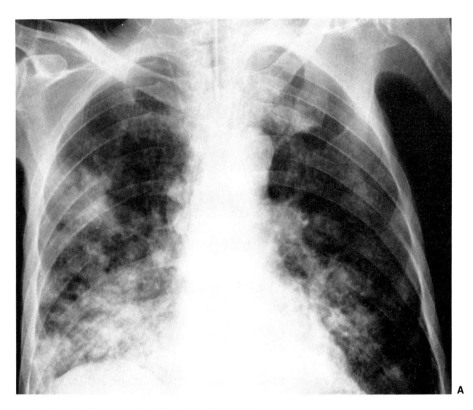

A

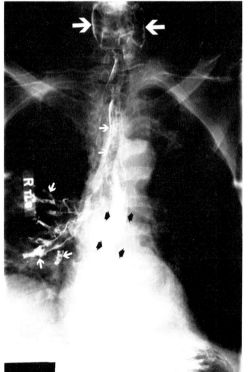

Figure 3–23. Diffuse aspiration pneumonitis. **A.** Infiltrates are primarily in dependent lower lobes. **B.** Esophagram (*black arrows*). Barium aspirated in tracheobronchial tree (*white medium and small arrows*); *large white arrows* demonstrate the pyriform sinuses in the hypopharynx.

B

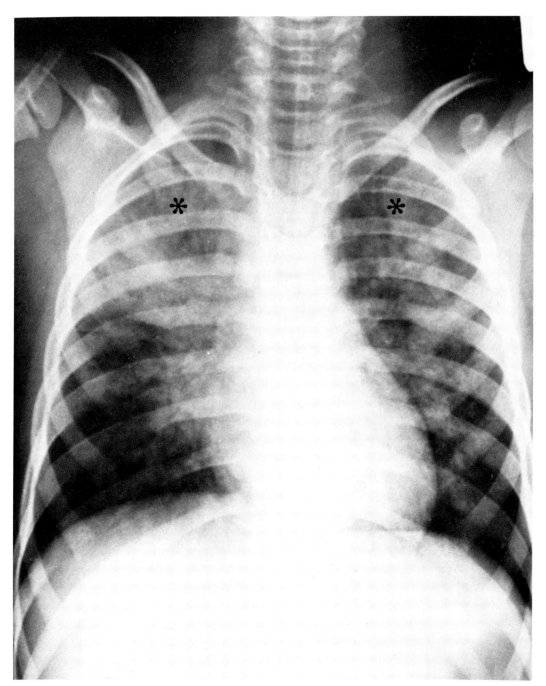

Figure 3–24. Aspiration pneumonitis involving upper lobes (*asterisks*).

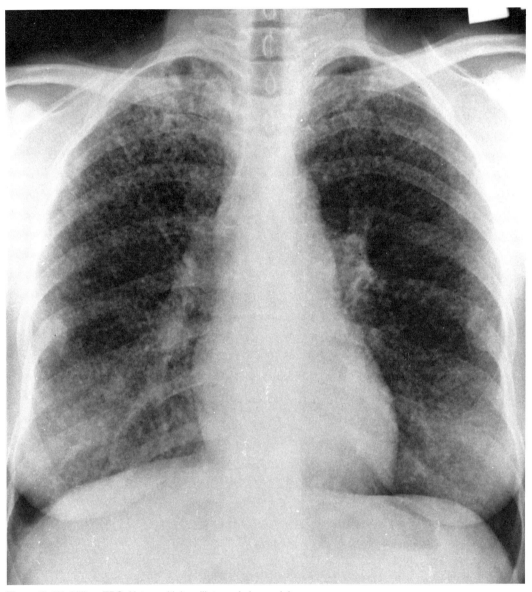

Figure 3–25. Miliary TBC. Note multiple millet seed size nodules.

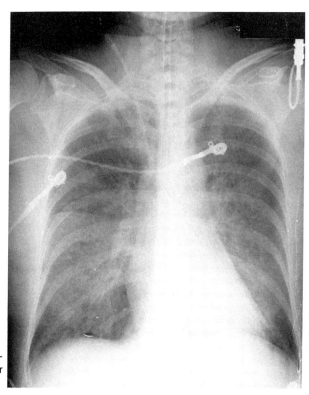

Figure 3–26. ARDS resulting from pneumococcal pneumonia. **A.** ARDS with diffuse alveolar disease.

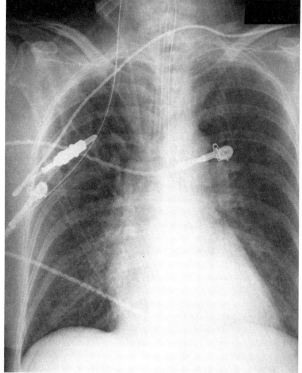

Figure 3–26B. Lung shows improved aeration after PEEP.

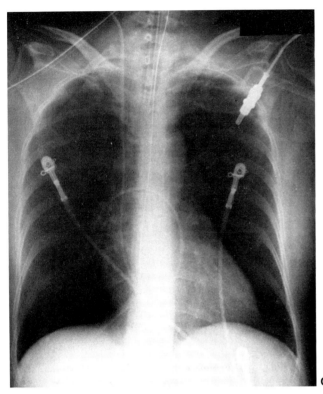

Figure 3–26C. Lung is well–aerated and shows no evidence of prior displayed alveolar disease. **D.** Reintubation required after removal from ventilatory support; note "recurrent" pulmonary edema.

C

D

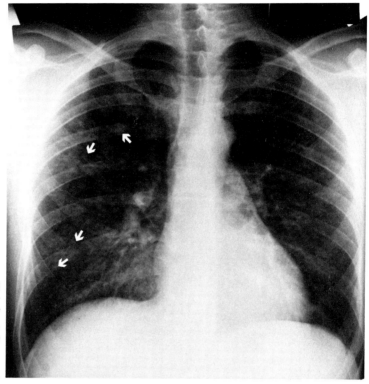

Figure 3–27. Diffuse toxic lung injury. **A.** Toxic inhalation of chlorine gas causes alveolar nodular changes (*arrows*) on right lung. **B.** Total resolution occurs two weeks later.

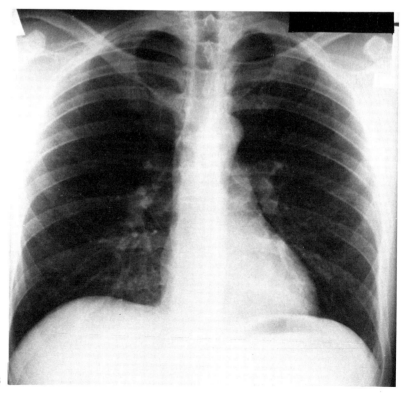

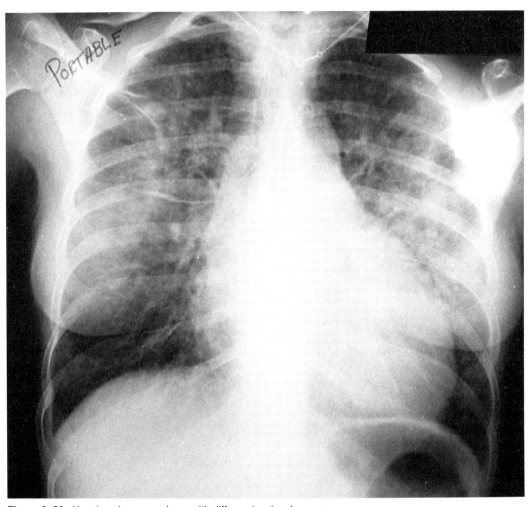

Figure 3–28. Uremic pulmonary edema with diffuse alveolar changes.

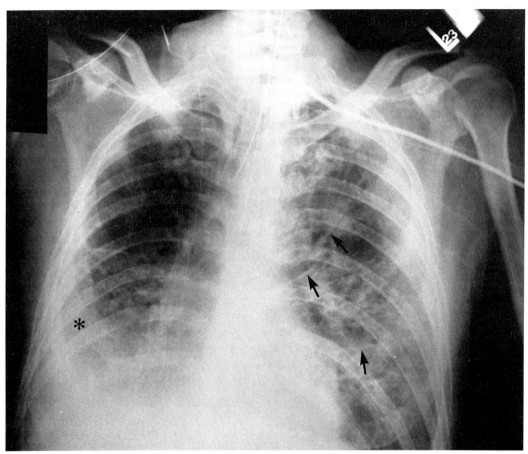

Figure 3–29. Lymphagitic metastases characterized by interstitial changes. Note Kerley's A lines (*arrows*) and right pleural effusion (*asterisk*).

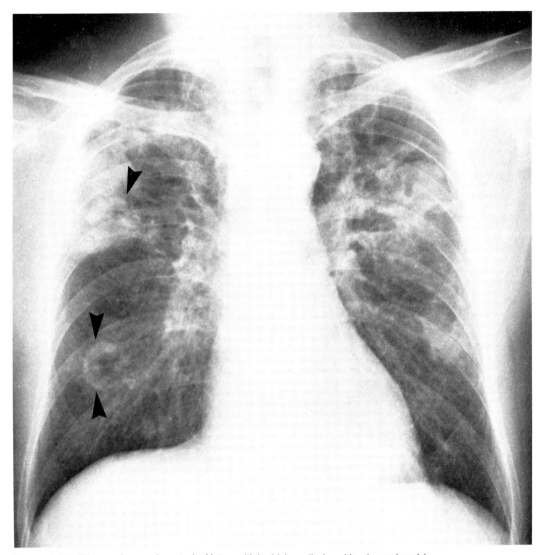

Figure 3–30. Wegener's granulomatosis. Note multiple thick–walled cavities (*arrowheads*).

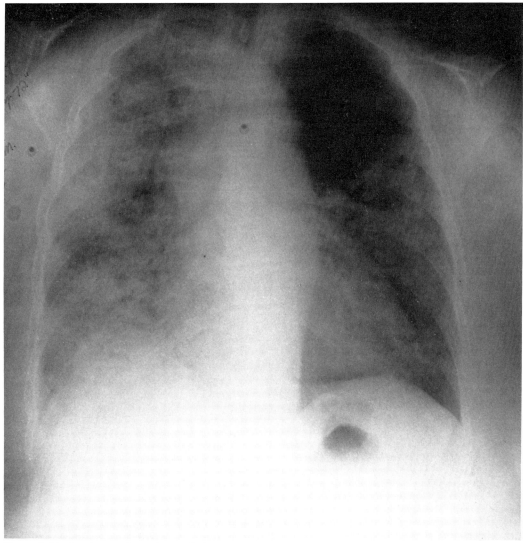

Figure 3–31. Goodpasture's syndrome. Pulmonary infiltrates are characterized by diffuse alveolar hemorrhage.

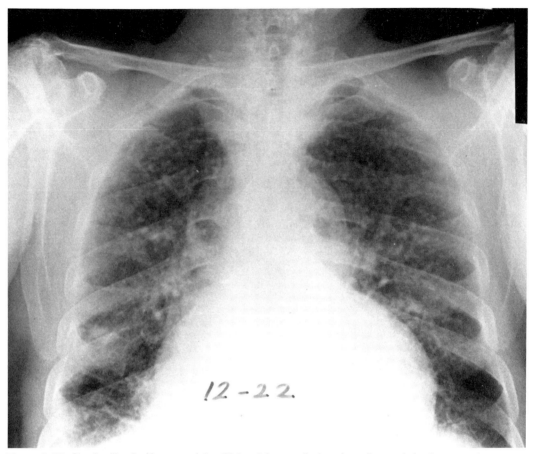

Figure 3–32. Simple silicosis. Numerous interstitial nodules are displayed; cardiomegaly is also present.

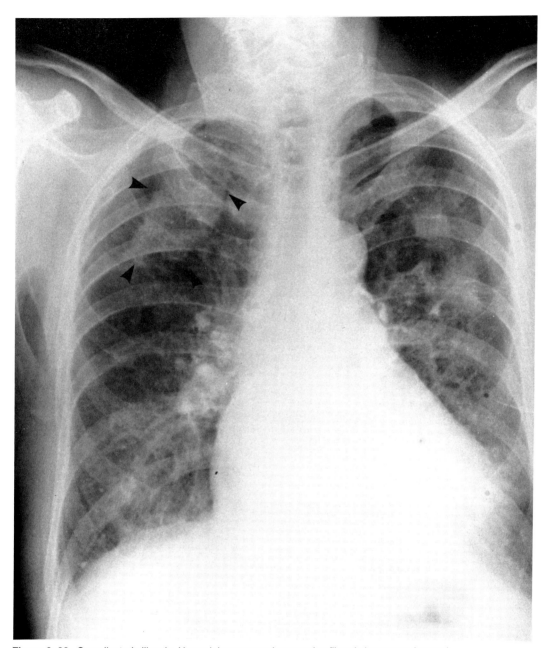

Figure 3–33. Complicated silicosis. Upper lobe progressive massive fibrosis is present (*arrows*).

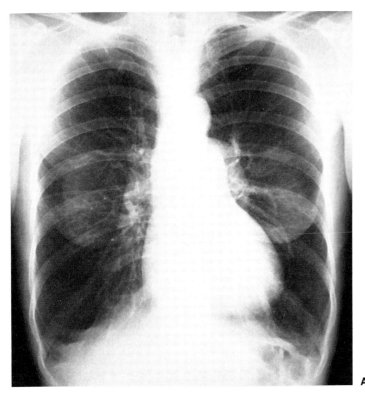

A

Figure 3–34. Decreased density. **A.** Emphysema with hyperlucent lungs. Note the depressed diaphragm. **B.** Depression of diaphragm seen on lateral film.

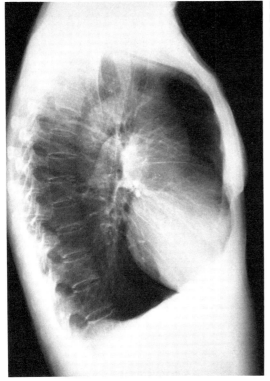

B

Chapter 4

Abnormal Air and Fluid

Lyle D. Victor, MD, *and David Yates*, MD

PNEUMOTHORAX

A collection of air between the visceral and the parietal pleura is known as a pneumothorax. Two important roentgenographic features are presented by a pneumothorax (Fig. 4–1). First, there are no pulmonary bronchovascular markings in areas of free intrathoracic air (*white circle*). Second, because air is less dense than the collapsed lung, a line of demarcation—the visceral pleura line (*white arrows*)—can be seen between the air and the lung. The *dark arrows* point out the medial border of the scapula.

Clinical comment on the size of a pneumothorax is based on the percentage loss of lung volume. It is, therefore, easy to conceptualize the greater-than-80% pneumothorax seen in Figure 4–1 when volume rather than area is considered. Knowledge of the pneumothorax percentage has clinical utility because a loss greater than 30% in selected clinical situations is used by some clinicians as sufficient reason for chest tube insertion to evacuate the air. Chest tubes may also be inserted for smaller pneumothoraxes in more critical situations, as might be seen in patients on mechanical ventilation.

Tension Pneumothorax

Occasionally, air enters the chest under conditions that impede its exit, thereby creating an ever expanding amount of intrathoracic gas under tension. Some experts believe that a "ball-valve" system is created, which allows air to enter but not to exit. This condition ultimately creates a pressure in the pleural space that is greater than the atmospheric pressure. The tension pneumothorax created is shown in Figure 4–2A. The *large white arrows* point to the totally collapsed lung; the *small black arrowheads* show the expanding air mass moving across the midline. The resultant mediastinal shift may cause compromise of the great vessels and consequent hypotension. The *small white arrows* show the relative increase in the size of the rib interspaces on the right in contrast to those on the left. This increase is due to hyperexpansion of the right hemithorax caused by the expanding pneumothorax. The flattened hemidiaphragm (*large white arrowhead*) seen in Figures 4–1 and 4–2A is another strong indicator of a tension pneumothorax. A chest tube placed anteriorly produced an immediate outward rush of air, relief of hypotension, and lung expansion (Fig. 4–2B). If the apex of the lung is nicked while placing subclavian or internal jugular catheters, it can cause a pneumothorax. A small one is shown in Figure 4–2C.

Not every faint vertical line on the chest roentgenogram indicates a pneumothorax. Skin folds are a common imitator. Consequently, exclusion of a pneumothorax requires identification of lung markings peripheral to the vertical line. The *white arrows* in Figure 4–3 point to skin folds; at the same time, faint pulmonary vessels can be seen just lateral to the tips of the *arrows*.

Mediastinal and Subcutaneous Air

Patients on ventilatory support are at high risk for barotrauma—especially if the lungs are poorly compliant as a result of inflammation or edema. Rupture of the alveoli can create interstitial air that may dissect medially along the bronchial connective tissue sheaths to enter the mediastinum and subcutaneous tissues. The child with adult respiratory distress syndrome (ARDS), whose chest film is shown in Figure 4–4, developed massive mediastinal air (*black arrows*) and subcutaneous air (*white arrows*). Because air can also dissect into the pleural space to form a pneumothorax (*white arrow*), the chest tubes shown in the x-ray film are necessary. Air may even enter the pericardial sac (*white circles*). Mediastinal air can also pass inferiorly into the retroperitoneum and peritoneal cavity.

The patient whose chest film is shown in Figure 4–5 was performing forceful Valsalva maneuvers during a vaginal delivery. Ruptured alveoli probably created the mediastinal and subcutaneous air (*arrows*).

Figure 4–6 demonstrates pneumopericardium which is pericardial air. This case was due to an esophageal carcinoma that perforated the pericardium.

On rare occasions, air can enter the vascular system to create an air embolus. This situation may occur during neurosurgical procedures in which the patient is in the upright position. In the critical care unit, vascular air entry may occur during catheter insertion or removal. Inasmuch as significant air emboli are often rapidly lethal, roentgenograms are difficult to obtain. The roentgenogram shown in Figure 4–7 was taken after a cadaver was injected with 300 mL of air—twice the commonly accepted lethal dose. The *asterisks* show air in the superior vena cava, right atrium, right ventricle, and pulmonary artery outflow tract. If an air embolus is suspected, the patient should be placed on the left side and in head-down position to trap the air in the right lateral aspect of the right ventricle or atrium so that it does not enter the pulmonary

circulation. There is also the possibility of evacuation by a catheter placed in these areas.

PLEURAL EFFUSIONS

A pleural effusion is a collection of fluid anywhere in the pleural space. In the upright roentgenogram, the presence of approximately 250 mL of fluid is necessary before radiographic visibility is possible. There are many etiologies of pleural fluid. The most common include transudates of body fluids (e.g., hypoalbuminemic states or congestive heart failure), exudates (e.g., pneumonias), malignant effusions, and bloody pleural fluid (e.g., trauma).

Figure 4–8A provides an example of a subtle pleural effusion. There is a slight amount of blunting of the right costophrenic angle (*arrow*) that indicates the presence of fluid. The upright lateral film is useful to identify pleural effusion because the visibility of the posterior costophrenic sulcus is improved (Fig. 4–8B). Ample fluid is also demonstrated on the right lateral decubitus film (Fig. 4–8C). Laying a patient on either side allows free fluid to float into a dependent position that obscures the lateral chest wall and actually forms a fluid level. Some radiologists feel that as little as 15 mL or less of fluid can be demonstrated by this technique. Lateral decubitus films can be obtained in the intensive care unit by placing a rigid plane (such as a cardiac board) underneath the patient before taking the roentgenogram.

Pleural effusion in the supine patient gravitates superiorly, laterally, and posteriorly (Fig. 4–9). Figure 4–9A shows the fluid obscuring the right hemidiaphragm, layering laterally, and forming superiorly an apical cap (*curved arrows*). The area of increased density in the mid right hemithorax is due to posterior fluid–layering (*asterisk*). Figure 4–9B is a cross–table lateral film of the same patient. The patient is supine and the x-ray tube makes its exposure in a horizontal direction. The *arrows* demonstrate that the pleural fluid does indeed layer posteriorly and superiorly. When the patient is too ill to lie on his side for a decubitus film, a cross–table lateral film can be obtained to determine the presence of pleural effusion.

Pneumonic Effusions

Pleural fluid generated secondary to the inflammation from a pneumonic process is known as a parapneumonic effusion. Figure 4–10 shows such an effusion in a patient with pneumococcal pneumonia. The *arrow* points to the meniscus of the effusion. The meniscus occurs often in cases of pleural effusions because fluid has a tendency to layer higher laterally than centrally.

Infected pleural fluid classically involves staphylococcal anaerobic or gram-negative pneumonias. When pleural fluid is associated with these pneumonias, empyema or pus in the pleural space should be suspected. The empyema classically is loculated or atypical in location (Fig. 4–11A). The sharp medial margin (*arrows*) indicates that the effusion in this patient with staphylococcal pneumonia is loculated. If the empyema contains air, the diagnosis is then quite definite. A thoracotomy tube (*large arrow*) was inserted in order to effect adequate drainage (Fig. 4–11B). The films demonstrate the classic appearance of an empyema consisting of loculated fluid and air.

If a prominent air–fluid level develops in a pneumonitis, a diagnosis of bronchopleural fistula must then be entertained (Fig. 4–12). A bronchopleural fistula is a direct connection between the bronchus and the pleural space allowing air to enter the pleural space directly. Chest–tube drainage is the treatment of choice for an empyema or a bronchopleural fistula.

Malignant Effusions

A malignant pleural effusion is shown in Figure 4–13A. The patient had adenocarcinoma. A thoracentesis was performed (Fig. 4–13B), but two hours later, the patient was short of breath because of reexpansion pulmonary edema (Fig. 4–13C). Acute pulmonary edema can develop in

a normal lung after removal of surrounding pleural fluid. The exact mechanism of this phenomenon is not well understood.

Subpulmonic Effusions

Fluid may collect in the space between the base of the lung and the diaphragm and may create a situation in which no distinct fluid level can be seen in the upright roentgenogram. Figure 4–14A shows some of the typical features of a subpulmonic effusion. The peak of the hemidiaphragm is typically moved laterally (*arrow*) by the fluid underneath. The decubitus film (Fig. 4–14B) verifies the presence of the fluid. The *white arrow* shows fluid tracking in the minor fissure. This patient had gallbladder surgery six days previously. About 60% of all upper abdominal surgeries show postoperative pleural effusions of some kind on the side of the surgery. The fluid collections are also called sympathetic effusions because they form in the hemithorax above the diaphragm, below which there is active disease.

Starvation-Induced Effusion

Pleural fluid frequently collects in patients who have been on mechanical ventilation for extended periods of time and who have inadequate nutrition. When the serum albumin decreases, it allows plasma oncotic pressure to fall and encourages intrapleural fluid collections. Figure 4–15A provides a typical example. Note the bibasilar haziness and the indistinct diaphragms—more prominent on the left than on the right. A left lateral decubitus film (Fig. 4–15B) was done at bedside and shows fluid layering (*arrowheads*).

Hemothorax

Blood, too, can cause pleural effusion. Figure 4–16 shows a patient who was over-anticoagulated with heparin and developed a large hemothorax.

Massive Effusion

A totally opacified hemothorax from pleural effusion can be caused by a ruptured esophagus, a dissecting aneurysm, or a neoplasm. An example of a malignant effusion is seen in Figure 4–17A. A large effusion of the left hemothorax is seen shifting the mediastinum to the right (*arrows*). An anterior chest tube with tetra-cycline instillation was placed for drainage and pleurodesis (Fig. 4–17B).

REFERENCES

Goodman LR: Review–Postoperative chest radiography. *AJR* 1980; 134: 533–546.

Tuddenham W: *Chest Disease Syllabus,* Philadelphia, American College of Radiology, pp 263–268.

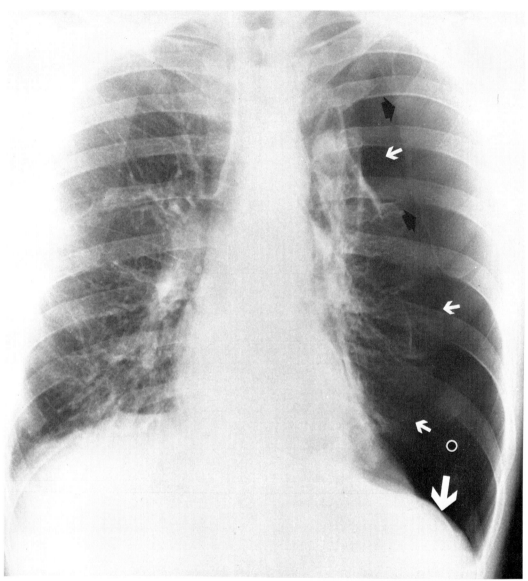

Figure 4–1. Tension pneumothorax. The scapula superimposes the chest (*black arrows*); the collapsed lung is outlined by visceral pleura (*small white arrows*); and the large amount of free pleural air without lung markings is visible (*circle*). The depressed left hemidiaphragm is a strong indicator of tension pneumothorax (*large white arrow*).

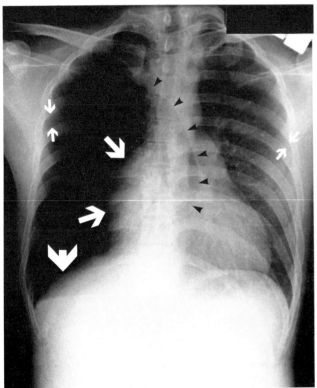

Figure 4–2. Tension pneumothorax. **A.** The right lung is totally collapsed (*large white arrows*); the medial margin of the pneumothorax has shifted the mediastinum to the left, placing it under pressure (*black arrowheads*); and the right hemidiaphragm is flattened (*large white arrowhead*). The *small white arrows* on the right demonstrate increase in rib interspace, indicative of volume increase from tension pneumothorax. This distance is considerably smaller on the left, shown by white arrows at the same inter space.

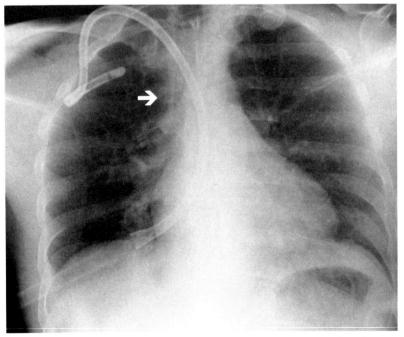

Figure 4–2B. Chest tube was inserted, pneumothorax was removed, and total expansion of right lung was effected. Note visibility of right-sided mediastinal structures that have shifted back to their original position (*white arrow).*

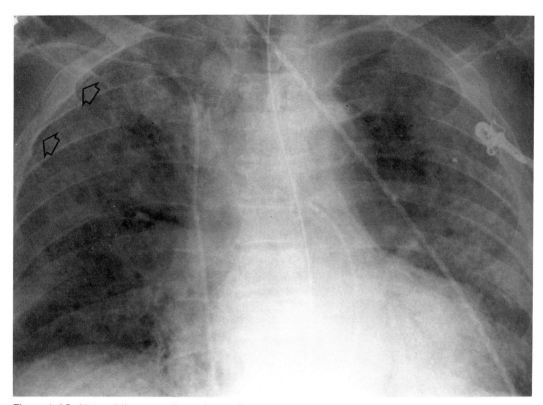

Figure 4–2C. Note subtle pneumothorax *(arrows).*

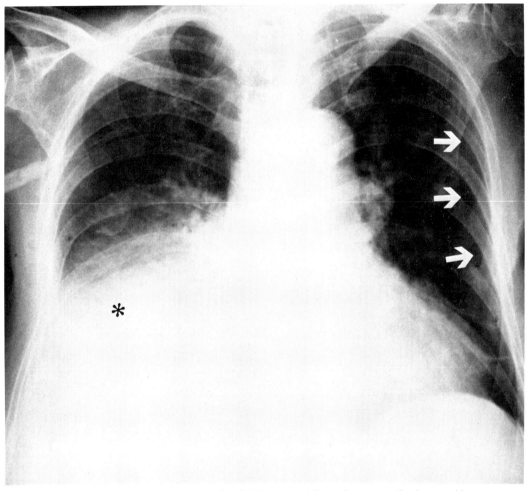

Figure 4–3. Skin fold imitating pneumothorax. Small white horizontal streaks representing lung markings are seen lateral to *white arrows*. *Asterisk* demonstrates a pleural effusion on the right.

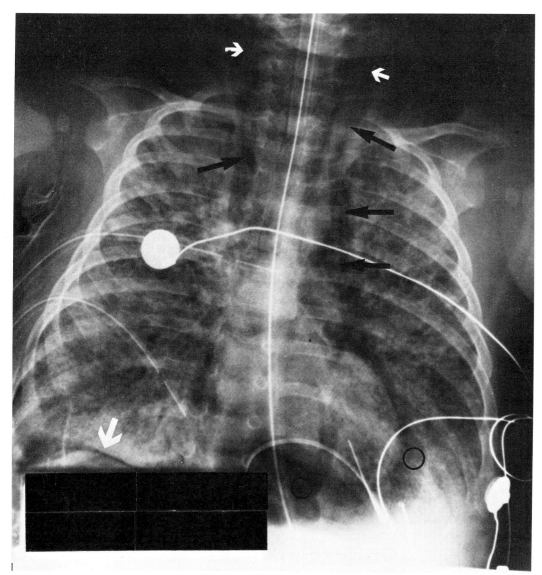

Figure 4–4 Barotrauma. Interstitial air has dissected into the mediastinum (*black arrows*). The fascial planes in the neck communicate with the mediastinum to cause the subcutaneous emphysema (*small white arrows*). Pericardial air (*circles*) may be caused by interstitial air in perivenous spaces dissecting into pericardium; *large white arrow* demonstrates pneumothorax.

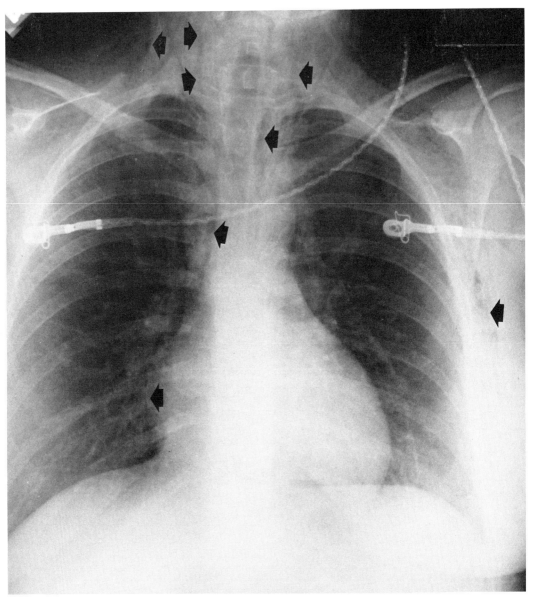

Figure 4–5. Mediastinal and subcutaneous emphysema (*black arrows*).

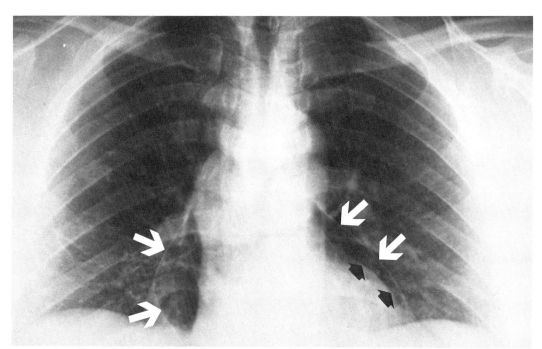

Figure 4–6. Pneumopericardium. *White arrows* demonstrate pericardium; epicardiac margin is sharply displayed (*black arrows*).

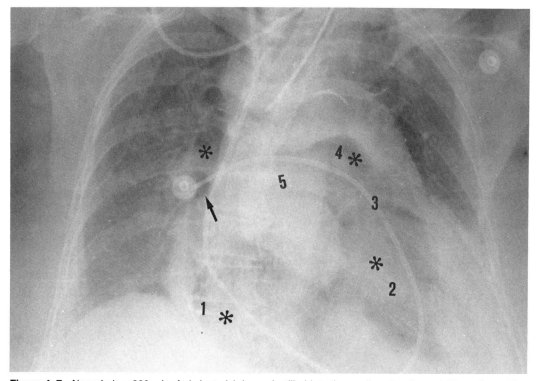

Figure 4–7. Air embolus. 300 mL of air (*asterisks*) was instilled into the cardiac chambers of this cadaver. The numbers indicate the following: 1, right atrium; 2, the right ventricle; 3, the main pulmonary artery; 4, the left pulmonary artery; 5, the right pulmonary artery. The *arrow* demonstrates the dilated balloon of the Swan–Ganz catheter.

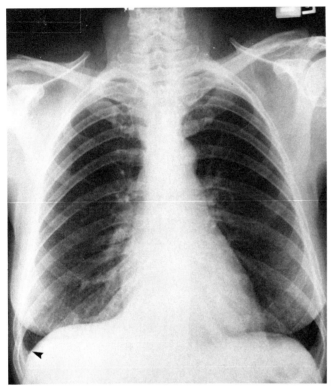

Figure 4–8. Small pleural effusion.
A. *Arrow* points to effusion.

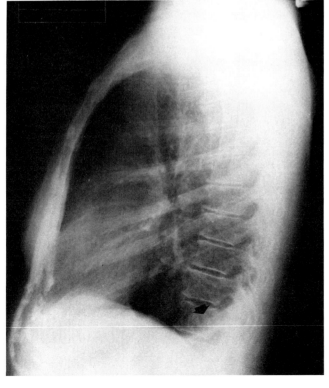

Figure 4–8B. Note fluid in the posterior costophrenic angle (*arrow*).

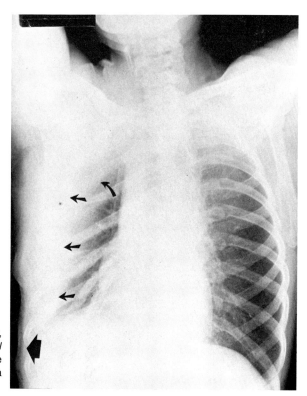

Figure 4–8C. In this right lateral decubitus film, *large arrow* indicates the right side is down; *small arrows* demonstrate the pleural fluid layering in the dependent position. Note medial border of scapula (*curved arrow*).

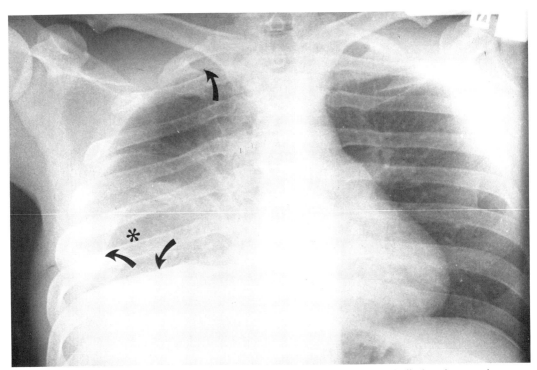

Figure 4–9. Pleural effusion in supine patient. **A.** *Curved arrows* indicate the pleural effusion; the *superior arrow* demonstrates apical pleural fluid cap. Increased parenchymal density (*asterisk*) represents posterior layering of pleural effusion.

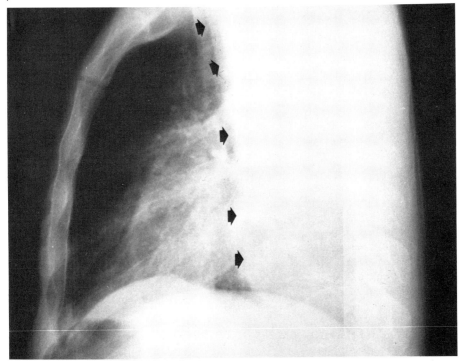

Figure 4–9 B. Cross-table lateral film demonstrates posterior layering of pleural effusion (*arrows*).

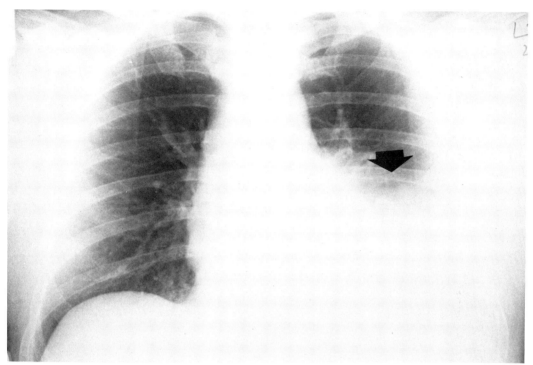

Figure 4–10. Parapneumonic effusion. *Arrow* points to meniscus of pleural effusion. Typically, these are laterally higher.

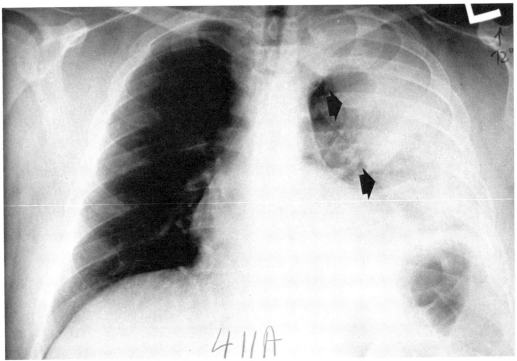

Figure 4–11. Empyema. **A.** Arrows denote sharp medial margin of effusion; indicates it is loculated.

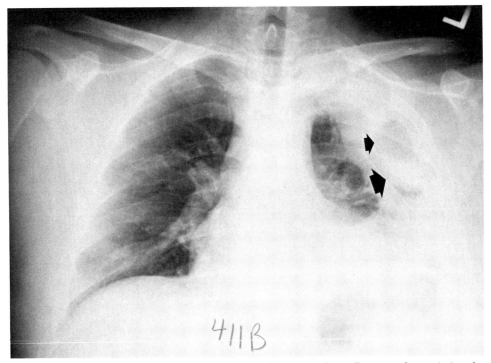

Figure 4–11B. Shows treatment by chest tube drainage (*large arrow*); smaller arrow demonstrates air typical of an empyema.

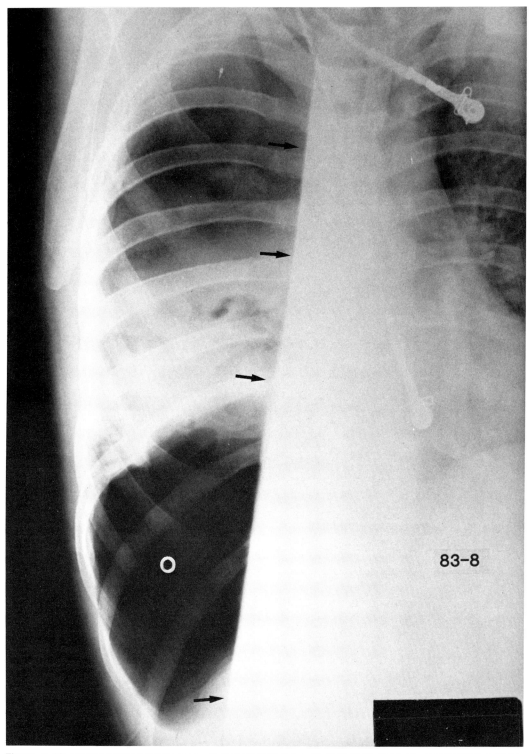

Figure 4–12. Bronchopleural fistula *(arrows)* demonstrate large air–fluid level. Free air, representing a pneumothorax, is denoted by the *white circle* in this left lateral decubitus film.

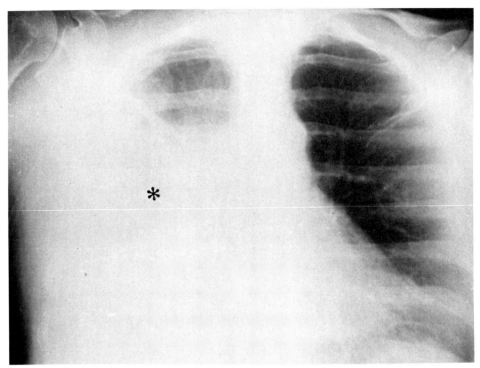

Figure 4–13. Postthoracentesis pulmonary edema. **A.** Note massive malignant pleural effusion on the right.

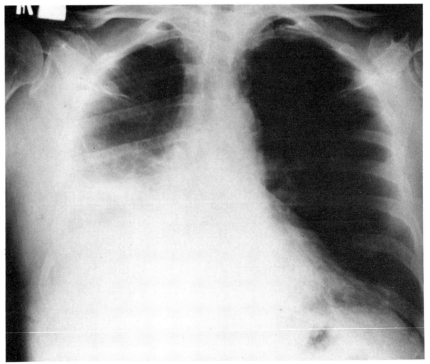

Figure 4–13B. Postthoracentesis film shows considerable improvement.

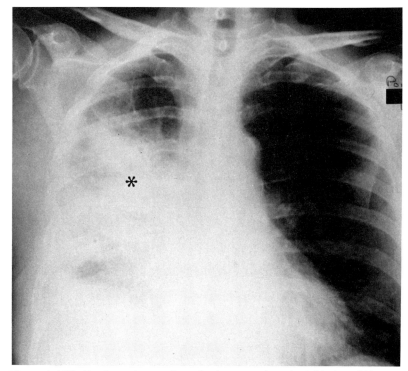

Figure 4–13C. Two hours later, unilateral pulmonary edema is visible (*asterisk*).

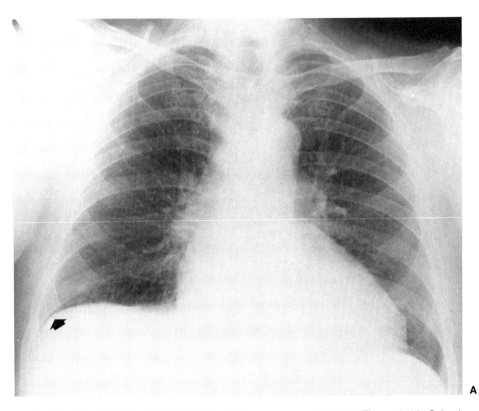

A

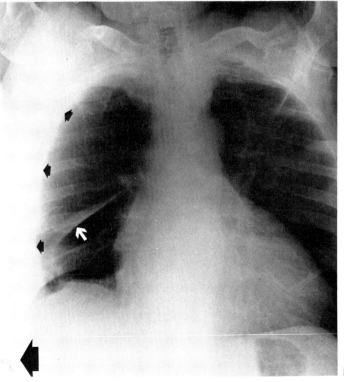

B

Figure 4–14. Subpulmonic effusion. **A.** Note lateral peaking (*arrow*). **B.** In this right lateral decubitus film, *large arrow* indicates right side down; *small arrows* demonstrate dependent fluid layering; *white arrow* demonstrates fluid gravitating to minor fissure.

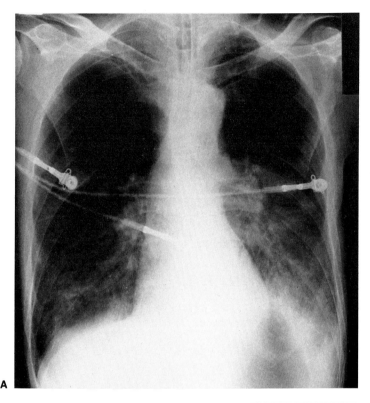

A

Figure 4–15. Hypoproteinemia. **A.** Bilateral obscuration of hemidiaphragm is due to pleural effusion. **B.** In this left lateral decubitis film, left side is down (*large arrow*). Note layering of effusion on left (*arrowheads*); the hemidiaphragm on the right is sharper because of dependent layering of fluid against the mediastinum.

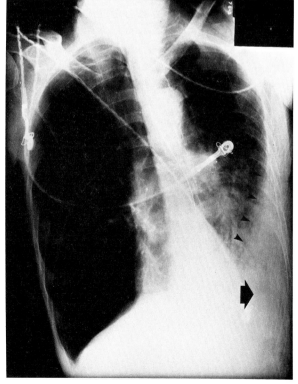

B

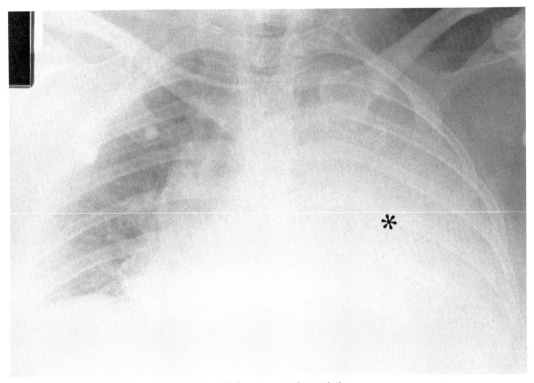

Figure 4–16. Large hemothorax on left (*asterisk*) from over-anticoagulation.

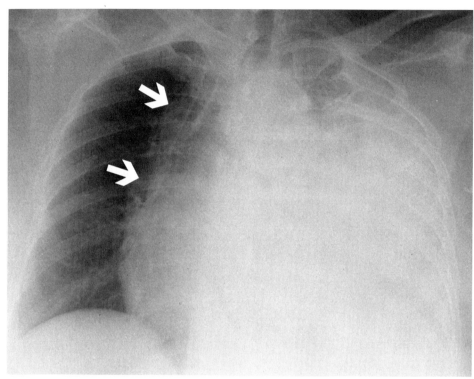

Figure 4–17. Massive left pleural effusion. **A.** Malignant effusion is pushing mediastinum to the right (*arrows*).

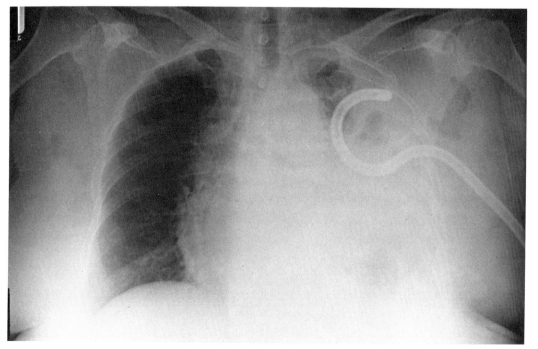

Figure 4–17B. Tube placed for drainage and pleurodesis and tetracycline instillation.

Chapter 5

Cardiovascular Disease

James I. Breckenfeld, MD, *Allen J. Stone*, MD,
and *Lyle D. Victor*, MD

Changes in the portable chest roentgenogram may provide the first signs of cardiac dysfunction. Early recognition of cardiovascular decompensation such as pulmonary vascular engorgement, ventricular enlargement, or pacemaker malplacement can be lifesaving. Complications of cardiovascular surgery are also frequently seen. The following are some examples of acute processes seen in the critical care unit or the coronary care unit.

CARDIOVASCULAR DECOMPENSATION

Congestive Heart Failure

The normal upright portable chest roentgenogram shows a relative paucity of vascular markings in the upper lobes because of gravitational effects. The chest film in Figure 5–1A demonstrates that the vessels in the upper lobes are smaller and fewer than those in the lower lobes (*large white arrows*). The vessels are also sharply delineated. The sharp contours of a peribronchial vessel are seen head on (*small white arrow*). When congestive heart failure (CHF) occurs, the heart becomes enlarged. Normally, the cardiac silhouette, measured at the heart's largest transverse diameter from the apex on the left (*large black arrow* on left) to the right heart margin, should be less than 50% of the widest thoracic diameter measured from the inner rib

margins (*open arrows*). In Figure 5–1B there is cardiac enlargement and the heart diameter is greater than 50% of the thoracic transverse diameter. During the initial stage of CHF there is an increase in the size and the apparent number of upper lobe vessels (*white arrows*). This cephalization can occur in the normal supine patient when the gravitational forces are applied more evenly. However, it is important to compare similar studies, whether they be supine or erect, to demonstrate alterations.

An increase in hydrostatic pressure in the lower lobe vasculature leads to a transudation of fluid into the interstitial space and causes a veiled appearance (*asterisk*) in the lower lobes (Fig. 5–1B). This increase in interstitial fluid causes a constriction in the lower lobe vessels and a shunting of blood to the upper lobe vasculature. The buildup of interstitial fluid causes an indistinctness of vasculature and also peribronchial cuffing (*small white arrow*) that represents increased interstitial fluid in the area adjacent to the bronchus.

The interstitial edema in Figure 5–1C is also manifested by horizontal lines, Kerley's B (*straight arrow*), in the outer half of the lung bases and by longer peripheral lines, Kerley's A (*curved arrows*), in the midlungs, extending to the hila. These lines represent fluid in the interlobular septa. Figure 5–1D demonstrates a magnified view of Kerley's lines.

Without treatment, the interstitial edema eventually leads to pulmonary alveolar edema accompanied by fluid pouring into the alveoli and causing 'a diffuse clouding of both lungs (Figs. 5–1E and 5–1F).

The butterfly pattern of pulmonary edema is classically seen in patients suffering from over-hydration and renal failure (Fig. 5–2). This pattern characteristically involves the perihilar and central portions, sparing the periphery. The pattern seen in cases of CHF, according to Milne, is one of diffuse involvement. Pleural effusions seen in Figure 5–3A can be a manifestation of left ventricular heart failure. Figures 5–3B and 5–3C show clearing of pleural effusions with treatment. When an isolated pleural effusion in the case of CHF is found, it is almost always on the right. The proclivity for fluid collection on the right in the case of CHF is an accepted fact. The etiology of this asymmetry is controversial. Bilateral pleural effusions found with a normal sized heart may not indicate heart failure and can be associated with hypoproteinemia, malignancy, and other conditions.

Mediastinal widening is seen in cases of CHF when this has progressed to right-sided decompensation (Figs. 5–4A and 5–4B).

Atypical Pulmonary Edema

Pulmonary edema may show an atypical appearance because of structural defects in the lungs. For example, Figures 5–5A through 5–5C demonstrate the progressive changes of CHF in a patient with emphysema. As CHF progresses, the greatest changes are in the right upper lobe; there, the least amount of emphysematous lung is destroyed. Pulmonary edema in emphysematous patients can masquerade as pneumonitis because of its atypical appearance.

Pseudotumor

Collections of fluid in interlobar fissures can mimic neoplasms when the real etiology is CHF (Fig. 5–6A; see also 5–3A.) The lateral roentgenogram can confirm the fissural location of these "masses" (Fig. 5–6B). These pseudotumors often disappear after adequate treatment of CHF (see Fig. 5–3), verifying the old maxim "diurese, then diagnose."

Valvular Heart Disease

Significant mitral valvular disease can result in distinctive roentgenographic findings. The patient shown in Figure 5–7 complained of dyspnea at rest. The chest x-ray film (Fig. 5–7A) shows increased density over the heart, the so-called "double density" that represents an enlarged left atrium typical of hearts with advanced mitral stenosis (*black arrows*). The *white arrow* demonstrates straightening of the left heart margin because of enlargement of the left atrial appendage. Figure 5–7B shows the left atriogram done at cardiac catheterization, which verifies the diagnosis of mitral stenosis with a large left atrium. These patients often develop atrial fibrillation, which leads to localized stasis of blood, thrombus formation, and systemic emboli. Figure 5–8A shows a long-standing calcified mural thrombus (*arrowheads*) in a patient with mitral stenosis. Notice the prominent central pulmonary arteries and the paucity of peripheral vasculature from the secondary pulmonary hypertension that so often develops in these patients. Figure 5–8B is a lateral view demonstrating an enlarged left atrium manifested by the posterior prominence of this chamber (*medium white arrow*). The right ventricular enlargement is demonstrated by its anterior encroachment on the anterior retrosternal air space (*large white arrow*). Because it does not extend behind the inferior vena cava at the level of the diaphragm (*small white arrow*), the left ventricle does not demonstrate enlargement on the lateral view.

Another valvular heart disease that exhibits distinctive roentgenographic findings is pulmonic valve stenosis (Fig. 5–9). In Figure 5–9A, the *smaller white arrow* denotes the dilated main and left pulmonary arteries—a result of post-stenotic dilatation. The *larger arrow* points to the enlarged right heart. This prominence of the right heart is seen in combination with dilatation of the right atrium, but it can occasionally be seen with an enlarged right ventricle. Structural enlargement of the right side occurs as a result of the increased cardiac work from pumping against a stenotic valve. The lateral view (Fig. 5–9B) demonstrates the enlarged right ventricle anteriorly encroaching on the anterior retrosternal air space (*large white arrow*). The *two smaller arrows* demonstrate the prominent main pulmonary artery. The *arrowheads* point to the prominent left pulmonary artery.

Ventricular Aneurysm

Just as an inadequate aortic wall can dilate to form an aneurysm, so, too, can a weakened left ventricular wall. Figure 5–10A shows left ventricular enlargement. The cardiac silhouette widened even further one month later after the patient developed an acute anterior myocardial infarction (Fig. 5–10B). The angular, lateral dilatation of the left ventricular wall is typical of a ventricular aneurysm. Intractable CHF and persistent ventricular arrhythmias are complications that may be encountered. If the complications are severe enough, a surgical aneurysmectomy may have to be performed.

Pericardial Effusion

The pericardial sac is a sheath of connective tissue surrounding the heart. Apparent cardiac enlargement can be seen if this space fills with fluid. Figure 5–11 shows a typical "water bottle" shaped heart—so called because of its flask-like shape when large amounts of pericardial fluid are present. Another example of cardiac silhouette enlargement from pericardial fluid is seen in Figure 5–12A. Occasionally verification of pericardial fluid can be made on the lateral roentgenogram. Figure 5–12B demonstrates abnormal separation of the epicardial and the mediastinal fat-pad stripes (*two large arrows*) by the enlarged white band of pericardial fluid (*smaller arrow*).

Pacemaker Complications

The normal position for a cardiac pacemaker electrode is in immediate contact with the right ventricular apex (Fig. 5–13A). Correct electrode positioning is verified on the lateral film (Fig. 5–13B), which demonstrates anterior placement in the apex of the right ventricle (*black arrowhead*).

This same patient developed the "twiddlers" syndrome, whereby she constantly turned the corpus of the pacemaker positioned underneath the skin surface in the upper anterior chest wall. The persistent rotation displaced the pacemaker electrode proximally into the right atrium (Fig. 5–13C and 5–13D; *arrows*). Another pacemaker complication is looping of the pacemaker wire in the right atrium (Fig. 5–14; *arrow*). The electrode is too medial in location and does not approximate the apex. Pacemaker malposition in the coronary sinus is shown in Figure 5–15A (*large arrow*); the pacemaker has turned upon itself at the tricuspid valve (*black arrow*) to pass into the coronary sinus. The lateral view (Fig. 5–15B) confirms the posterior positioning of the pacemaker in the coronary sinus. Because the coronary sinus also passes to the left, the electrode is sometimes positioned on the left, mimicking the location of the right ventricle. Usually, however, the catheter positioned on the left points superiorly toward the left shoulder.

A broken pacemaker is shown in Figure 5–16 (*large arrows*). The roentgenogram shows a supplementary pacemaker wire in place and outlined by the *small arrowheads*. A newer type pacemaker, which is achieving popularity, is an atrioventricular sequential pacemaker that paces in a progressive fashion: electrodes in the right atrium pace first, and electrodes in the right ventricle pace second (Fig. 5–17). This type of pacing is preferred by many clinicians—especially in situations of ventricular dysfunction—because it has the potential, through an "atrial kick," to increase cardiac output.

Aortic Aneurysm

The aorta is a thick-walled elastic vessel, which must tolerate the constant systemic pressure of the left ventricular output. Isolated areas of weakness may manifest themselves as aneurysmal dilatation. The danger of an aortic aneurysm is rupture, shock, and exsanguination. Figures 5–18A through 5–18C show progressive aortic aneurysmal dilatation of the descending aorta occurring over a two-year period in a patient with arteriosclerotic heart disease. An aneurysm of the ascending aorta is shown in Figure 5–19B. The patient had a previous aortic valve replacement (Fig. 5–19A). Figure 5–19C, a computerized tomography (CAT) scan, demonstrates the massive aneurysmal dilatation of the aortic root (*arrows*).

An aortic aneurysm may also be the result of blunt trauma. Figure 5–20 demonstrates the result of a steering wheel injury that occurred when the victim's vehicle struck an oncoming vehicle. Figure 5–20A demonstrates widening of the mediastinum (*arrowheads*), obscuration of the aortic knob, and a left apical cap. All of these conditions are due to an extensive mediastinal hematoma. The apical extrapleural region communicates with the mediastinum and allows blood to pass into this region. With the above findings, it is imperative to exclude a laceration of the aorta. Figure 5–20B is a thoracic aortogram demonstrating a traumatic aneurysm (*small wide arrows*) in the aortic isthmus—the region beyond the left subclavian artery (*thin arrow*), which is attached to the ligamentum arteriosum. This location is classic for the deceleration injury of the aorta that is associated with steering wheel injuries. The *small wide arrows* display the traumatic aneurysm.

Coarctation of the Aorta

Congenital coarctation of the aorta is associated with several distinctive roentgenographic findings. Figures 5–21A and 5–21B demonstrate rib-notching (*arrows*), which occurs when the prominent intercostal arteries bypass the coarctation. The stenotic aorta (coarctation), usually occurs distal to the origin of the left subclavian artery (Fig. 5–21C; *curved arrows*). The left subclavian artery and the segment of aorta between it and the coarctation are dilated (*medium arrows*). There is also poststenotic dilatation of the aorta (*large arrow*) beyond the coarctation (*curved arrow*). This condition creates "two moguls with a valley between." Figure 5–21D demonstrates these findings more clearly on an aortogram. Coarctations are associated with hypertension, biscuspid aortic valves, and left ventricular failure.

Pulmonary Vascular Disease

One of the most common and difficult diagnostic problems is pulmonary embolus. Typically, the chest film is negative, although basilar atelectasis (see Chapter 3) or pleural effusion may be encountered. Because of vascular occlusion, vascular markings may be reduced segmentally or regionally. This regional pulmonary oligemia is called Westermark's Sign. In cases in which there has been a complete loss of blood supply, pulmonary infarction can occur; they appear as localized infiltrates at the periphery of the lung at the pleural margins (Figs. 5–22A and 5–22B). A rounded lateral density known as a Hampton's hump is a roentgenographic sign of pulmonary infarct. Figure 5–23A shows a nuclear lung scan of another patient and demonstrates a segmental perfusion defect typical of pulmonary embolus. The *arrow* points to the perfusion defect. There is a distinct segmental defect in the area of the posterior segment of the right upper lobe that persists on most of the standard views. Figure 5–23B shows a normal scan performed two weeks after heparin therapy was instituted. A pulmonary angiogram may be necessary when a strong clinical suspicion of pulmonary embolus exists and the lung scan is indeterminate because of underlying pulmonary disease. Figure 5–24 demonstrates an embolus (*arrow tip*) creating a typical hyperlucent defect in the contrast material.

Because pulmonary angiography poses an increased risk of morbidity secondary to the required pulmonary artery catheterization, a less invasive, yet accurate, method of demonstrating pulmonary embolus is needed. A promising new technique, digital subtraction angiography, may fill this role. The dye is injected into only a peripheral vein. Enhancement of the pulmonary vasculature is effected by computer subtraction of the surrounding densities.

Traumatic Fat Embolus

In some cases of skeletal trauma, particularly to the lower extremities or pelvis, fat from bone marrow may enter the venous circulation and ultimately lodge in the pulmonary parenchyma.

Patchy infiltrates or the more diffuse alveolar edema of adult respiratory distress syndrome (ARDS) may appear. This disorder is usually treated with ventilatory support and oxygenation along with proper treatment of the trauma (Figs. 5–25A and 5–25B). The radiologic findings are usually delayed until 24 to 48 hours after the trauma.

Pulmonary Hypertension

Elevated blood pressure in the pulmonary circulation may occur as a primary, idiopathic event. It is most often seen in young women (Figs. 5–26A and 5–26B). Pulmonary hypertension may occur also as a secondary phenomenon to cardiovascular pathology. Many diffuse lung diseases that cause widespread vascular damage to the lung have been associated with pulmonary hypertension (e.g., chronic obstructive pulmonary disease and recurrent pulmonary emboli). Acute and chronic arterial hypoxemia is associated with pulmonary vascular constriction and secondary pulmonary hypertension. Cardiac diseases such as atrial septal defect (Fig. 5–27) can eventually result in pulmonary hypertension accompanied by reversal of a left to right shunt as the hypertension increases. Figure 5–27 also demonstrates prominent peripheral pulmonary arteries, which would not be a classic finding for pulmonary hypertension. Figures 5–28A and 5–28B demonstrate pulmonary hypertension resulting from mitral valve disease. Roentgenographically, pulmonary hypertension is manifested by central blood vessel prominence and a relative paucity of peripheral vessels, well-demonstrated in the above figure.

COMPLICATIONS OF CARDIAC SURGERY

Valve Replacement

The normal position of a prosthetic cardiac valve is shown in Figure 5–28A. The *large arrow* points to a tricuspid valve replacement; the *middle-sized arrow* shows the mitral valve replacement; and the *thin arrow* shows the aortic

valve replacement. Large pseudotumors (*asterisk*) due to fluid in the fissures are present along with bilateral basilar pleural effusions. A lateral view is presented in Figure 5–28B.

The patient shown in Figure 5–29 had a porcine mitral valve replacement (*large arrowhead*). His mediastinal drainage tube developed blockage of its side holes (small arrowhead), which resulted in a superior mediastinal widening from a loculated hematoma (*white arrows*). The *black arrow* points to the tip of a pericardial drainage tube. In the case of another patient who had mitral valve replacement (Fig. 5–30; *large arrowhead*), a stent broke off and lodged in the splenic artery (*small arrowhead*). The *white arrow* points to an endotracheal tube placed too high in the trachea. An open mitral commissurotomy was performed on the patient shown in Figure 5–31. Subsequent bleeding into the pericardium led to pericardial tamponade. The resultant bulging cardiac contours are shown by the *white arrows*.

The Balloon Pump

Mechanical support of blood pressure in patients in cardiogenic shock and in the perioperative period of cardiac surgery can be effected by percutaneous aortic balloon counterpulsation. The proper position of the balloon's tip if it is to generate adequate cardiac output, is at the level of the aortic arch (Fig. 5–32). The tip of the catheter has been placed too cephalad into the left subclavian artery in the patient shown in Figure 5–33.

Coronary Artery Bypass Surgery

Complications that result from the median sternotomy performed during open-heart surgery may be visible by roentgenography. Figures 5–34A and 5–34B show a sternal dehiscence. Figure 5–34A is the chest film made immediately postoperatively; the sternum is intact. Figure 5–34B is a film made shortly after one of the sternal sutures broke (*large arrow*), allowing separation of the sternum (*arrowheads*). The site of separation partially superimposes the trachea. Markers for the bypassed coronary arteries are shown by the *thin arrows*.

Metal markers may be placed at the time of bypass surgery to denote the exact location of bypass grafts (Fig. 5–35A; *black arrow*). This patient had a foreign-body reaction to one of the markers and developed a secondary infection accompanied by abscess formation. A fistula developed from the sternal surface to the anterior mediastinum and graft origin. The swollen edematous soft tissue is marked by the *white arrow*. Figure 5–35B shows contrast outlining the fistulous tract and the abscess in the retroster-nal region (*arrow*). The *arrowhead* demonstrates contrast at the infected graft site.

A hydropneumopericardium is shown in Figures 5–36A and 5–36B. This patient walked into the hospital a few weeks after coronary artery bypass surgery. The origin of the air in this instance was thought to be air from a cutaneous fistula. The *large arrows* demonstrate an air-fluid level.

REFERENCE:

Milne, EN: Correlation of physiologic findings with chest roentgenology. *Radiol Clin of North Amer* 1973; 11:17–47.

Figure 5–1. Cardiovascular changes accompanying CHF. **A.** Negative chest. *Large white arrows* demonstrate sharply delineated vasculature; lower lobe vessels are more plentiful and larger than upper lobe vessels. *Small white arrow* shows thin wall of peribronchial vessel; *black arrows* display widest diameter of normal size heart; *clear arrows* show widest diameter of chest; metallic clips are from previous surgery. **B.** CHF, same patient. Heart is enlarged; its transverse diameter is greater than 50% of the widest transverse chest diameter. *White arrows* demonstrate prominent upper lobe vessels; peribronchial cuffing is shown by *smaller white arrow;* note veiled effect of interstitial edema (*asterisk*).

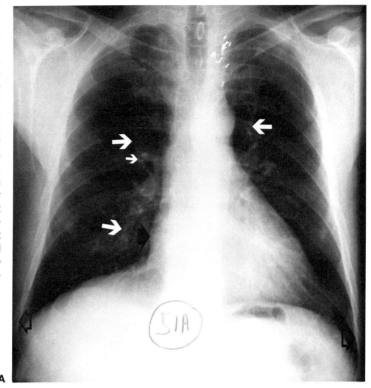

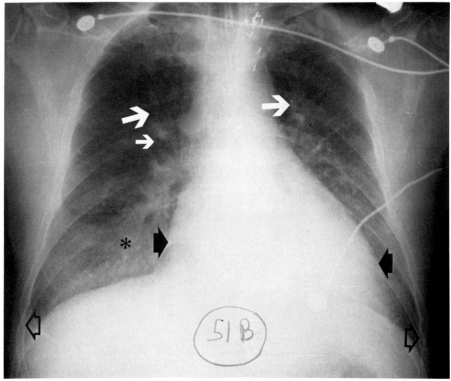

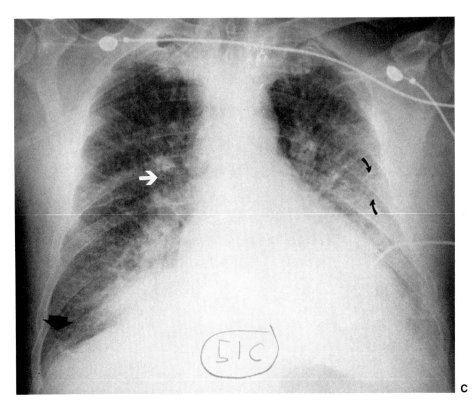

C

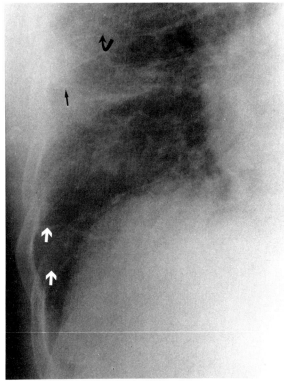

Figure 5–1C. Interstitial pulmonary edema. *Wide arrow* displays Kerley's B Lines; *curved arrows* demonstrate Kerley's A lines; note increased peribronchial cuffing (*thin straight arrow*). **D.** Note Kerley's B lines (*lower arrows*), Kerley's A lines (*straight black arrow*), minor fissure (*curved arrow*).

D

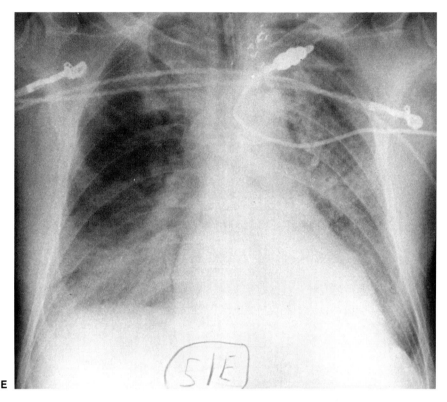

E

Figure 5–1E. Note progression to pulmonary alveolar edema with diffuse alveolar parenchymal changes. **F.** Pulmonary alveolar edema in another patient.

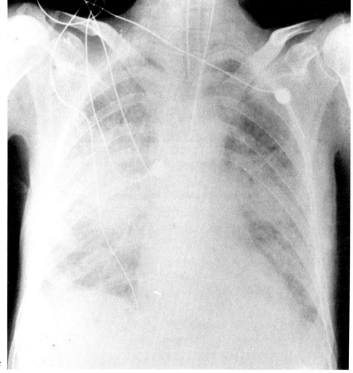

F

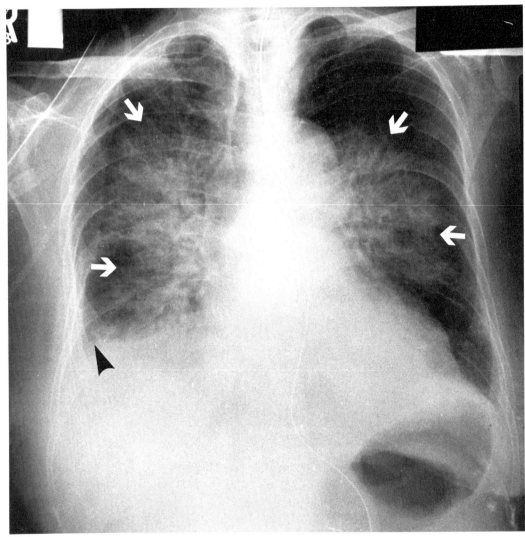

Figure 5–2. Butterfly or batwing appearance of pulmonary edema in patient with renal failure. *White arrows* demonstrate central involvement; note right-sided pleural effusion (*black arrowhead*).

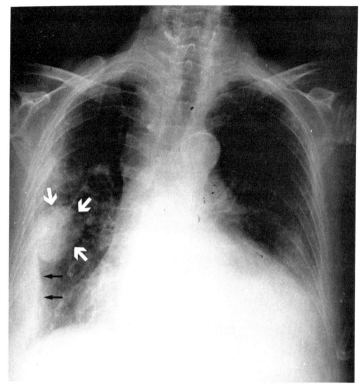

Figure 5–3. Bilateral pleural effusions with cardiac enlargement. **A.** Right-sided pleural effusion demonstrates lateral layering (*black arrows*); loss of hemidiaphragm on the left with hazy appearance of lower left lung suggests pleural effusion on left; note pseudotumor in minor fissure (*white arrows*). **B.** Note after treatment decreasing minor fissure fluid (*white arrow*) and right-sided pleural effusion (*black arrow*).

A

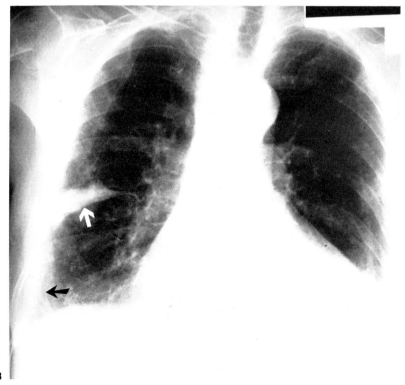

B

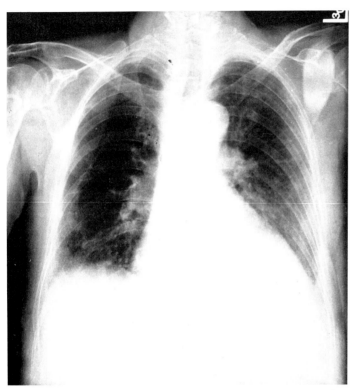

Figure 5–3C. Minor fissure has regained normal appearance. Note also improvement in the pleural effusions.

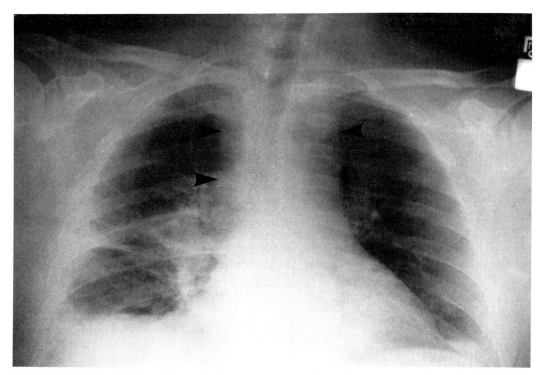

Figure 5–4. CHF. A. Widening of the mediastinum, due to systemic vascular engorgement, is seen with right-sided heart decompensation (*arrowheads*).

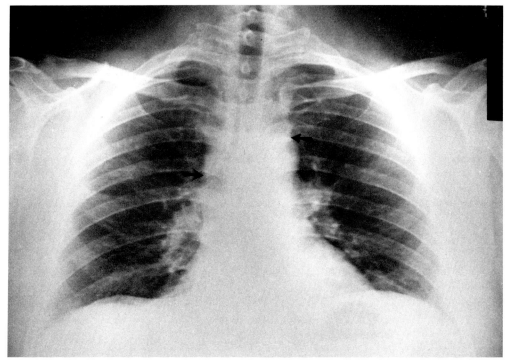

Figure 5–4B. Mediastinal width has decreased with treatment.

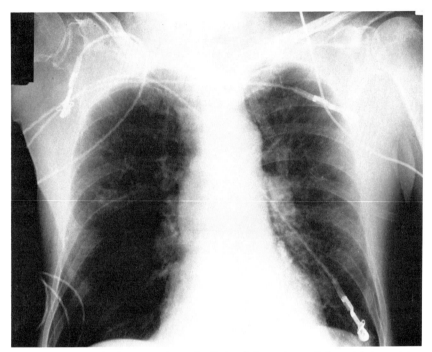

Figure 5–5. Atypical pulmonary edema. **A.** Patient is in respiratory failure; right lower lobe is hyperexpanded.

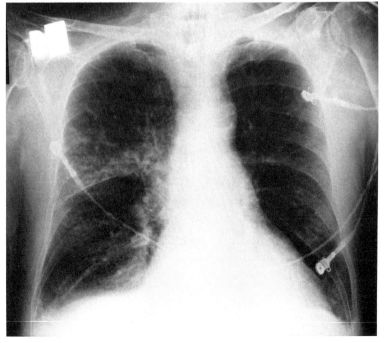

Figure 5–5B. Note pulmonary vascular congestion and interstitial edema in right upper lobe.

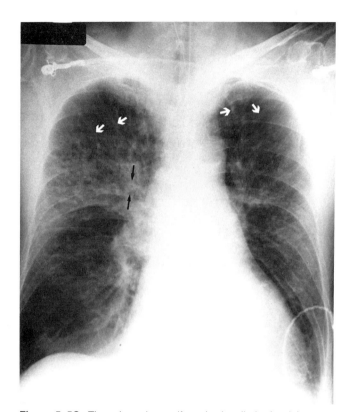

Figure 5–5C. The edema is manifested primarily in the right upper lobe. Note peribronchial edema or cuffing (*black arrows*) and vascular congestions (*white arrows*). The smallest amount of change is demonstrated in the right lower lobe, which has the greatest underlying structural change resulting from emphysema.

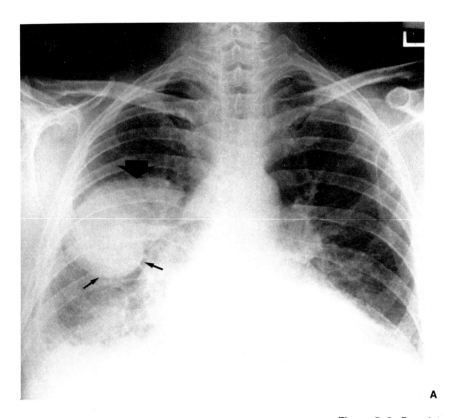

A

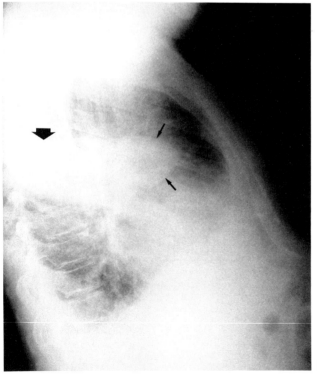

B

Figure 5–6. Pseudotumor seen in patient with congestive heart failure. **A.** *Small arrows* point to the minor fissure; *large arrow* denotes major fissure. **B.** Lateral roentgenogram demonstrates fluid-filled minor fissure (*small arrows*) extending posteriorly into major fissure (*large arrow*).

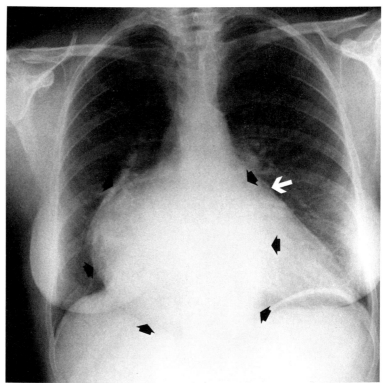

Figure 5–7. Mitral valve disease. **A.** Note large left atrium creating a double density (*black arrows*); straight left margin of the heart can be seen with enlarged left atrial appendage (*white arrow*).

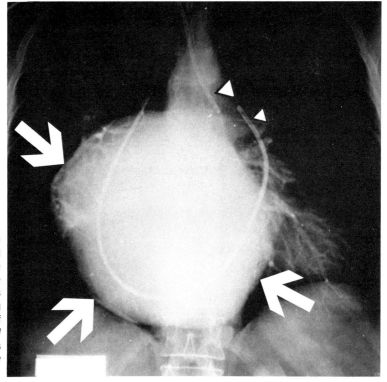

Figure 5–7B. Large obstructed left atrium is filled with contrast material (*white arrows*); *large white arrowhead* demonstrates catheter in the descending thoracic aorta for left side of heart catheterization; *small white arrowhead* displays catheter in main pulmonary artery at its bifurcation.

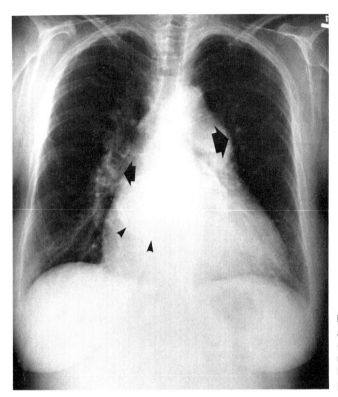

Figure 5–8. Calcified mural thrombus. **A.** Calcified left atrial mural thrombus (*arrowheads*) is in patient with mitral stenosis; *large arrow* points to large main and left pulmonary arteries; *small black arrow* points to enlarged right pulmonary artery.

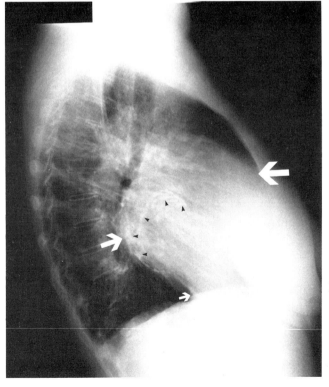

Figure 5–8B. Same patient, lateral view: *Large white arrow* demonstrates large right ventricle; *medium white arrow* points to posterior margin of large left atrium; *small white arrow* points to inferior vena cava. Left ventricle is not shown posterior to this point, and so it is not enlarged. Note calcified left atrial mural thrombus (*arrowheads*).

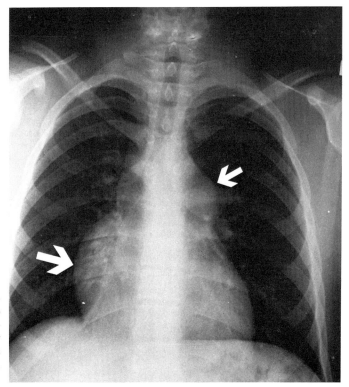

Figure 5–9. Pulmonary valvular stenosis. **A.** *Small white arrow* points to large main pulmonary artery in continuity with enlarged left pulmonary artery; *large white arrow* demonstrates large right heart that, in this instance, represents enlarged right ventricle.

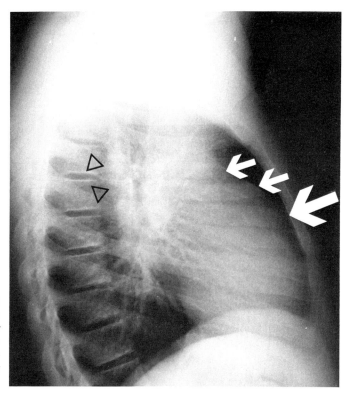

Figure 5–9B. Same patient, lateral view: *large white arrow* points to enlarged right ventricle; *two smaller arrows* display enlarged main pulmonary artery; *two arrowheads* point to posterior margin of enlarged left pulmonary artery.

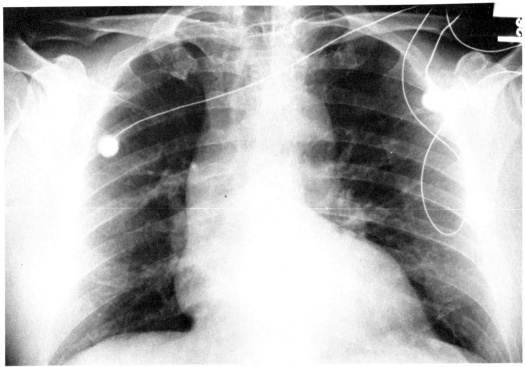

Figure 5–10. Weakened left ventricular wall. **A.** Enlargement of cardiac silhouette is due to left ventricular enlargement.

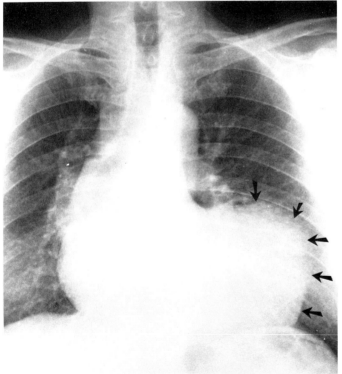

Figure 5–10B. One month later. Note ventricular aneurysm (*arrows*) after a myocardial infarction.

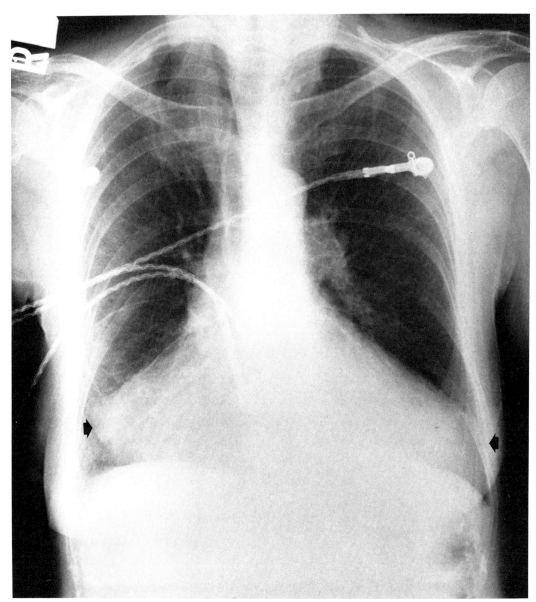

Figure 5–11. Pericardial effusion. *Arrows* display wide lower portion of the cardiac silhouette.

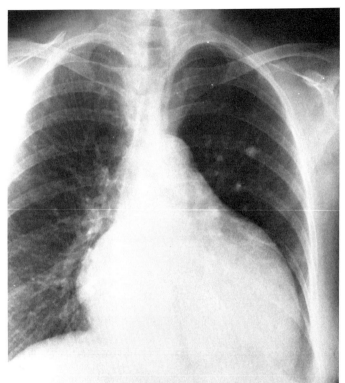

A

Figure 5–12. Pericardial effusion. **A.** Appearance of effusion is less characteristic than that shown in Figure 5–11. **B.** Same patient, lateral view: *posterior large arrow* demarcates the epicardial fat; *anterior large arrow* demarcates the mediastinal fat; *small arrow* demonstrates the white band of pericardial fluid between the fat densities.

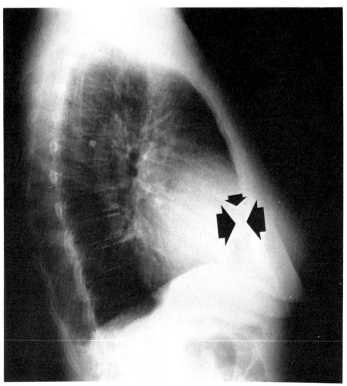

B

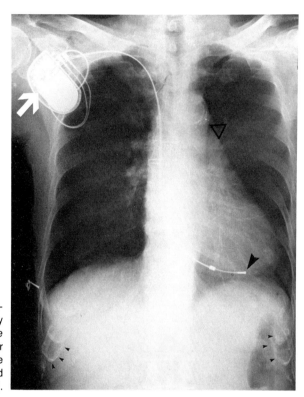

Figure 5–13. Normal position of pacemaker electrode. **A.** Cardiac pacemaker electrode is properly positioned at cardiac apex in right ventricle (*large black arrowhead*). Note that pacemaker power unit is buried in soft tissue (*white arrow*). Note calcified costal cartilage (*small arrowheads*) and calcification of the aortic arch (*white arrowhead*).

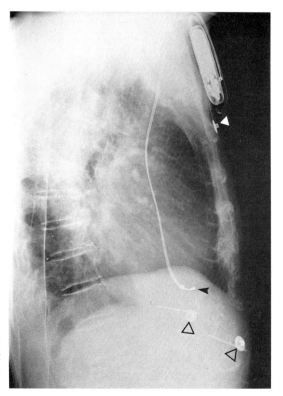

Figure 5–13B. Lateral view. Note that proper position of electrode is anterior to right ventricular apex (*black arrowhead*); *white arrowheads* point to EKG monitoring leads on skin surface.

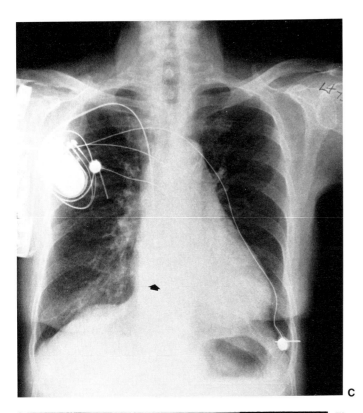

C

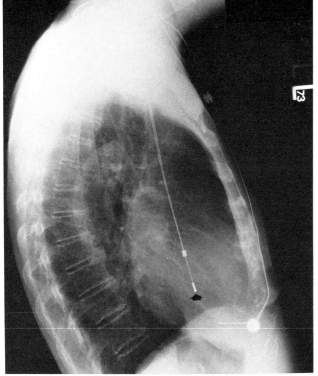

Figure 5–13C. Twiddler's syndrome has displaced electrode. **D.** Note that electrode has been manipulated into the right atrium (*arrow*).

D

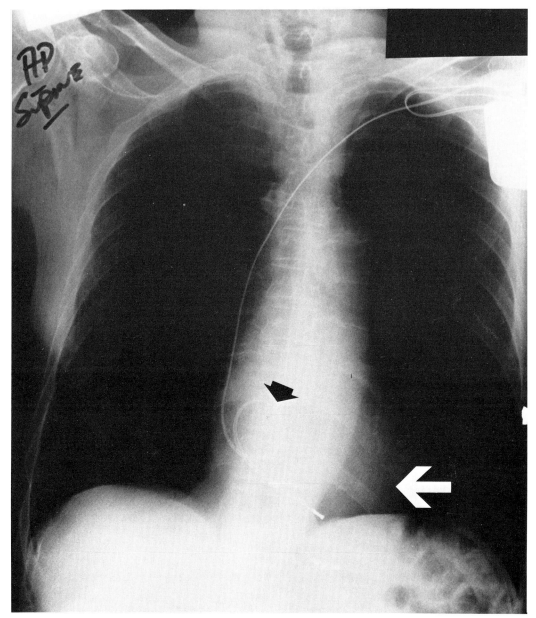

Figure 5–14. Looping of pacemaker wire in right atrium. Electrode appears to be too close to medial in location, not at the apex (*white arrow*).

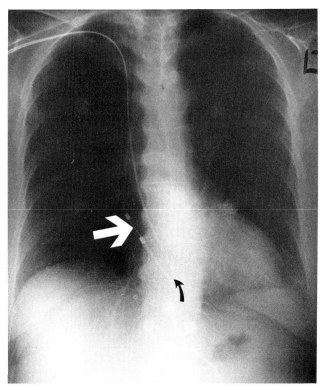

Figure 5–15. Pacemaker malposition. **A.** Pacemaker electrode is coiling at tricuspid valve (*black arrow*) to pass retrograde into the right atrium and coronary sinus (*white arrow*).

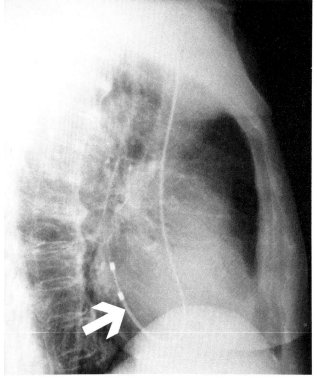

Figure 5–15B. Lateral view confirms posterior position of electrode in coronary sinus (*white arrow*).

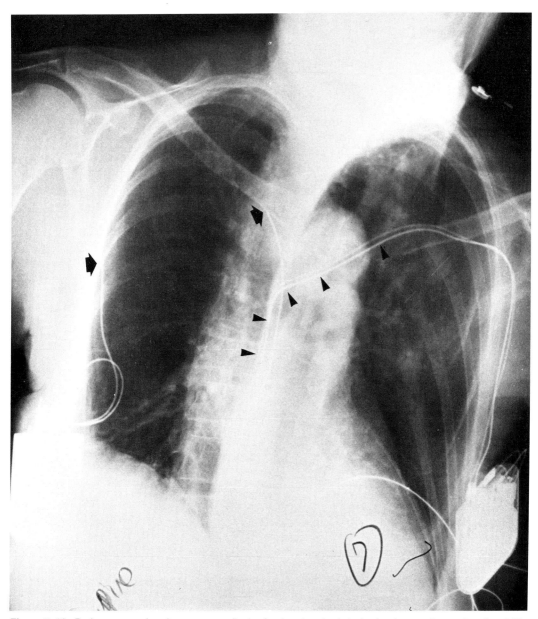

Figure 5–16. Broken pacemaker. *Large arrows* display fractured ends of electrode wire; *small arrowheads* point to replaced electrode wire.

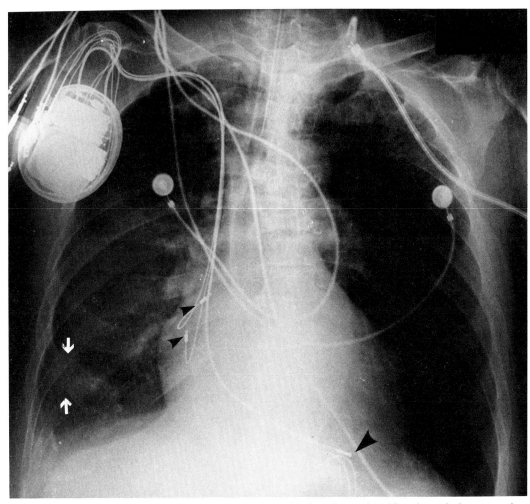

Figure 5–17. Sequential pacemaker. Note two atrial electrodes (*small arrowheads*) and ventricular pacemaker electrode (*large arrowhead*). Recent rib fractures shown by *white arrows.*

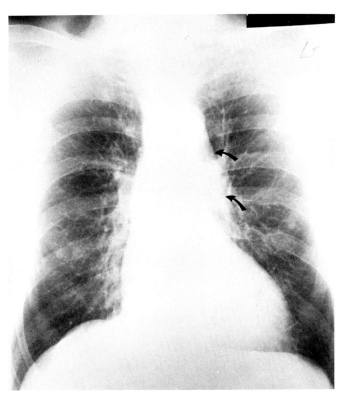

Figure 5–18. Aortic aneurysmal dilatation. **A.** Note elongation of descending thoracic aorta (*curved arrows*).

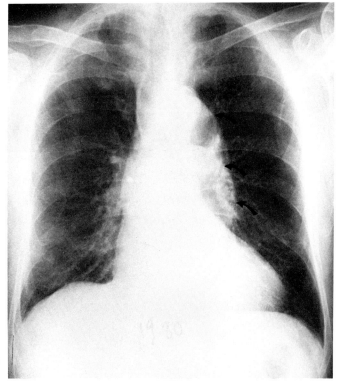

Figure 5–18B. Film displays aneurysm of aorta (*curved arrows*).

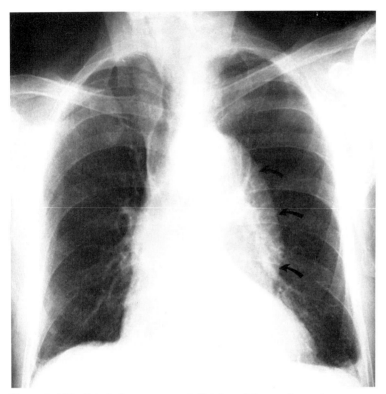

Figure 5–18C. Note further aneurysmal dilatation of descending aorta.

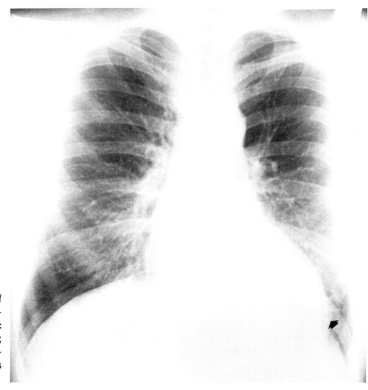

Figure 5–19. Aneurysm of ascending aorta. **A.** Note left ventricle enlargement before aortic valve surgery for aortic stenosis; apex of heart (*arrow*) points downward to left, which is seen in cases of left ventricular enlargement.

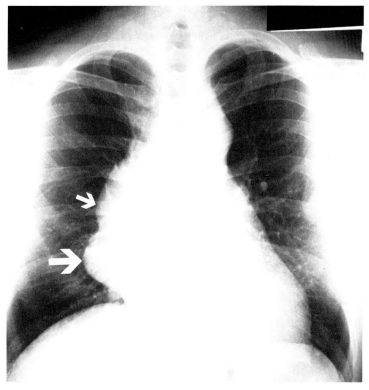

Figure 5–19B. Large aneurysm of ascending aorta caused lateral displacement of right atrium (*large white arrow*); *small white arrow* points to aneurysm.

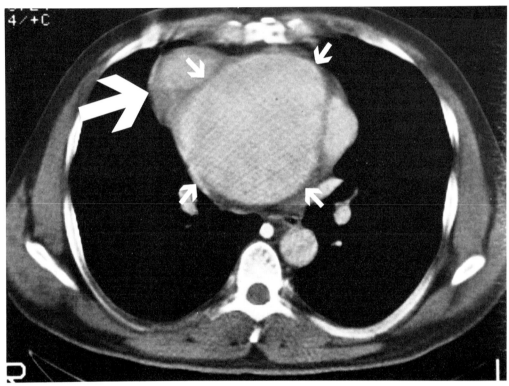

Figure 5–19C. CT scan shows large aneurysm of ascending aorta outlined by *small white arrows; large white arrow* demonstrates anterolateral displacement of right atrium.

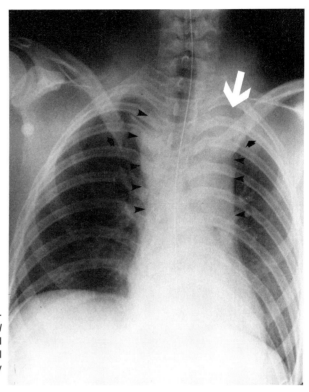

Figure 5–20. Traumatic mediastinal hematoma. **A.** Note widening of mediastinum (*small arrowheads*); white arrow displays left apical extrapleural cap; *black arrows* point to bilateral clavicular fracture; aortic knob is obscured by hematoma.

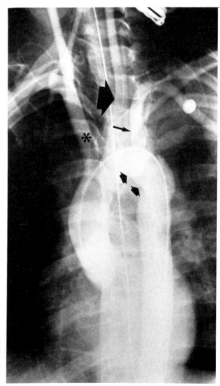

Figure 5–20B. Thoracic aortogram demonstrates traumatic aneurysm of aortic isthmus (*wide arrows*); thin arrow points to left subclavian artery; *asterisk* displays the innominate or brachiocephalic artery; note left common carotid artery (*large arrow*).

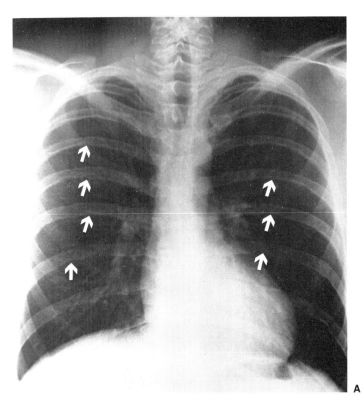

A

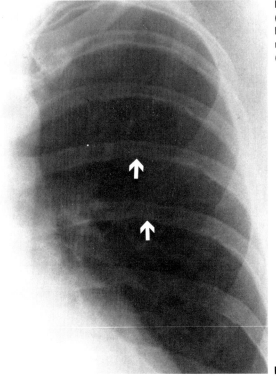

Figure 5–21. Coarctation of aorta. **A.** Rib notching (*arrows*) is due to prominence of intercostal arteries bypassing coarctation. **B.** Magnified view shows rib-notching classically on the inferior surface. (*arrows*).

B

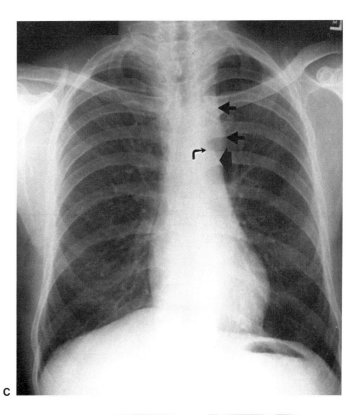

C

Figure 5–21C. *Two long arrows* display dilated subclavian artery and aorta just proximal to the coarctation (*curved arrow*); wide arrow displays poststenotic aorta. **D.** In this thoracic aortogram, *two long white arrows* point to dilated left subclavian artery and aorta proximal to the coarctation (*curved arrow*); note poststenotic aortic dilatation (*large arrow*).

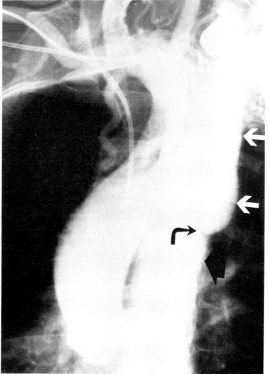

D

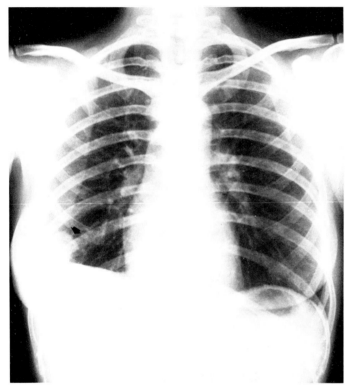

Figure 5–22. Pulmonary infarction. **A.** Note Hampton's hump (*arrow*).

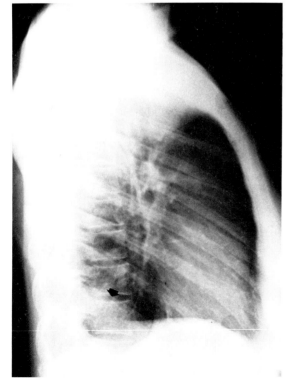

Figure 5–22 B. Lateral view displays its peripheral location.

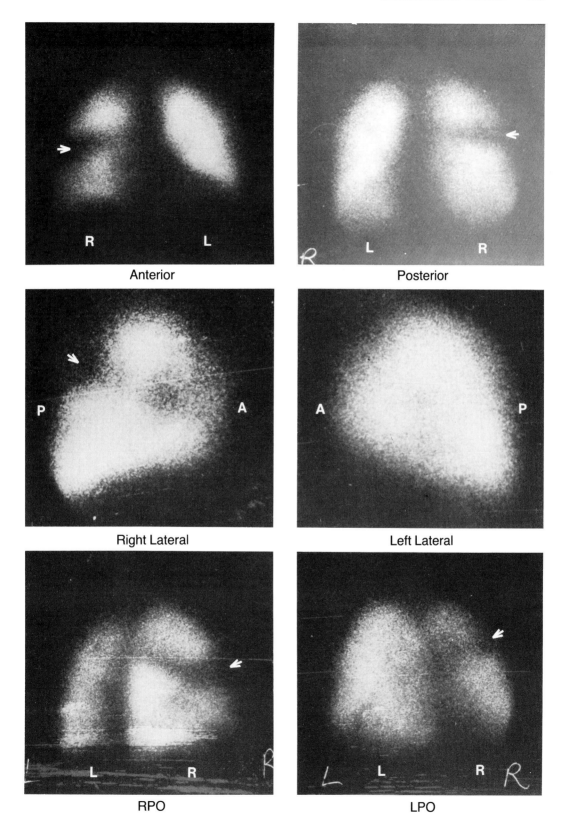

Anterior

Posterior

Right Lateral

Left Lateral

RPO

LPO

Figure 5–23. Lung scan. **A.** *Arrow* points to a perfusion defect of the posterior segment of the right upper lobe caused by a pulmonary embolus.

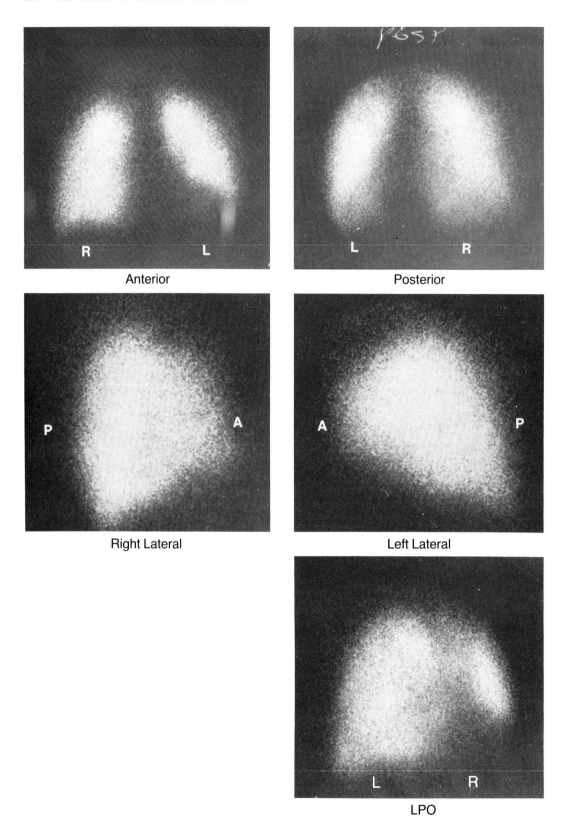

Anterior

Posterior

Right Lateral

Left Lateral

LPO

Figure 5–23B. Two weeks later, there is resolution of embolus; scan is normal.

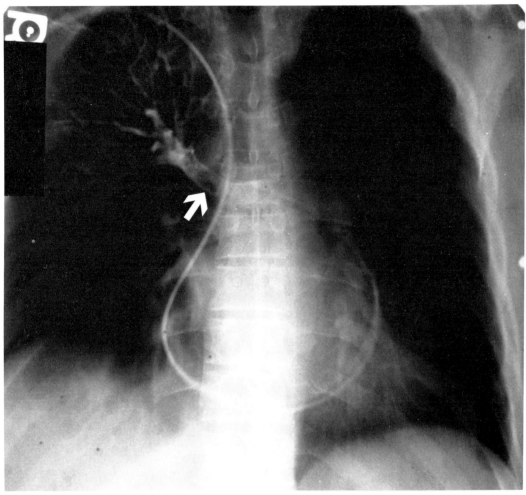

Figure 5–24. Pulmonary angiogram. Demonstrates an embolus (*white arrow*) in the right upper lobe pulmonary artery.

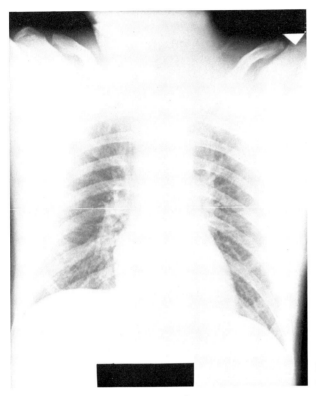

Figure 5–25. Fat embolus. **A.** Admission roentgenogram shows no abnormality.

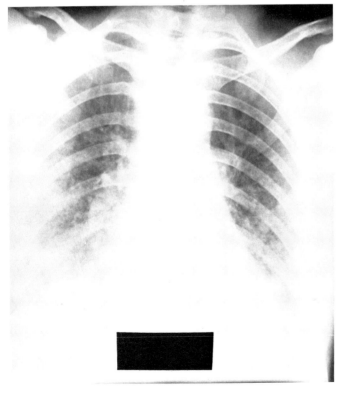

Figure 5–25B. Two days later, diffuse infiltrate due to fat emboli can be seen primarily in lower lung fields.

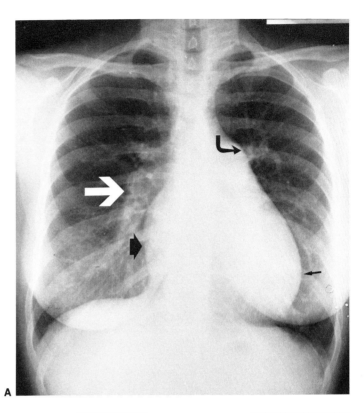

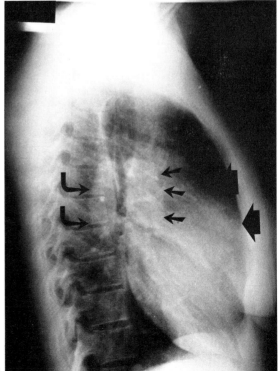

Figure 5–26. Primary pulmonary hypertension. **A.** Rounding and elevation of left margin of heart (*thin straight arrow*) are clues to right ventricular enlargement; *large black arrow* points to prominent right atrium; *curved black arrow* displays prominent main pulmonary and left pulmonary artery; large right pulmonary artery is displayed by *large white arrow*. **B.** *Two large arrows* point to the right ventricular outflow tract leading into the prominent main pulmonary artery; note prominent right pulmonary artery (*three straight arrows*) and prominent left pulmonary artery (*two curved arrows*).

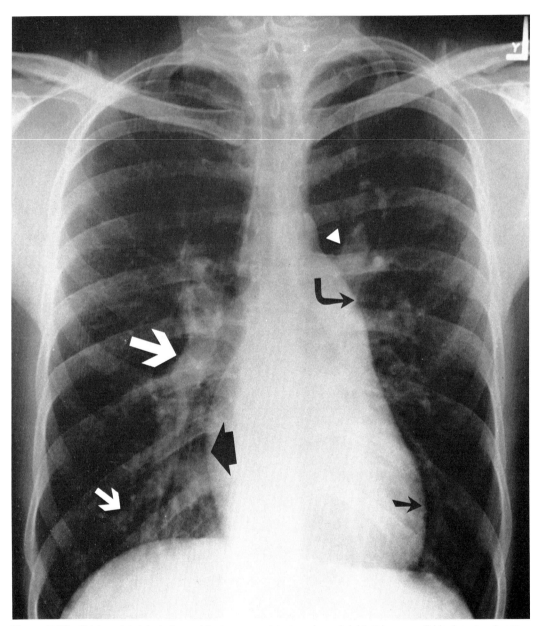

Figure 5–27. Atrial septal defect. *Large black arrow* points to enlarged right atrium; *small black arrow* denotes elevation of cardiac apex indicative of right ventricular enlargement. Note prominent main pulmonary artery (*curved arrow*), prominent left pulmonary artery (*white arrowhead*), large right pulmonary artery (*large white arrow*), and prominent peripheral pulmonary artery (*small white arrow*).

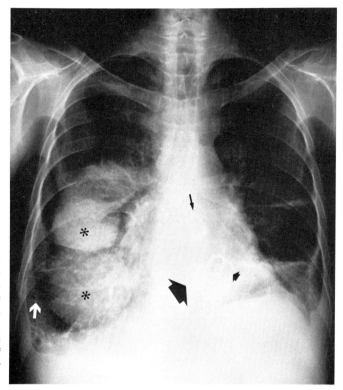

Figure 5–28. Prosthetic cardiac valves. **A.** *Thin arrow,* points to aortic valve prosthesis in central, high position; *medium-sized arrow,* mitral valve prosthesis–low on left; *large arrow,* tricuspid valve prosthesis–low and close to midline; *asterisks,* indicate large pseudotumors; *white arrow,* Kerley's B lines. Note paucity of blood vessels secondary to pulmonary hypertension.

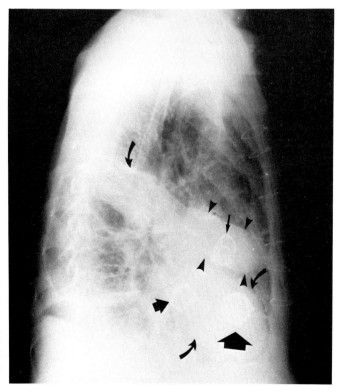

Figure 5–28B. Lateral view: *thin arrow* demonstrates superior position of aortic valve; *medium arrow,* posterior, low position of mitral valve; *large arrow,* anterior, inferior position of tricuspid valve. Note pseudotumor of major fissure (*curved arrows*) and pseudotumor of minor fissure (*arrowheads*).

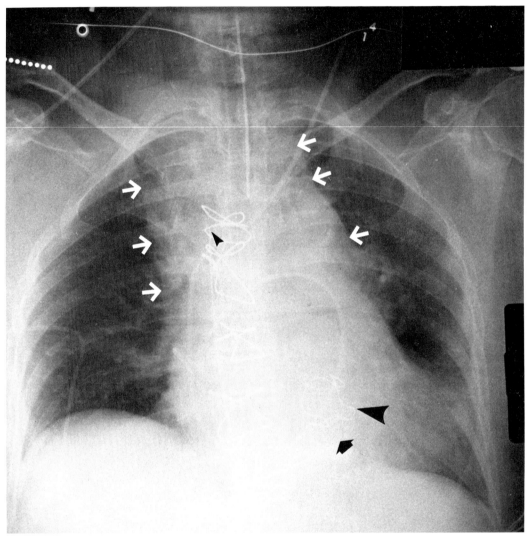

Figure 5–29. Porcine mitral valve replacement (*large arrowhead*). Note pericardial drainage catheter (*black arrow*), mediastinal drainage catheter (*small arrowhead*), and mediastinal hematoma (*white arrows*).

Source: Phillip Cascade, MD.

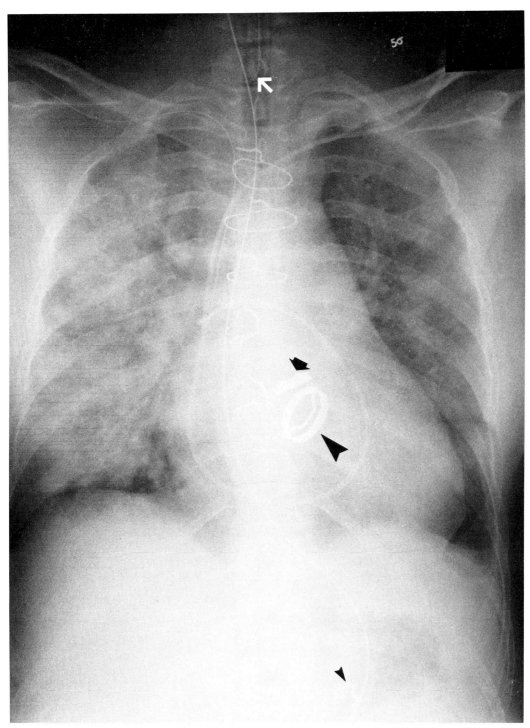

Figure 5–30. Postmitral valve insertion. *Large arrowhead* indicates mitral valve prosthesis; *small arrowhead,* metallic stent dislodged from valves passing through systemic circulation to the splenic artery; *large black arrow,* aortic valve prosthesis; *white arrow,* high position of endotracheal tube.

Source: Phillip Cascade, MD.

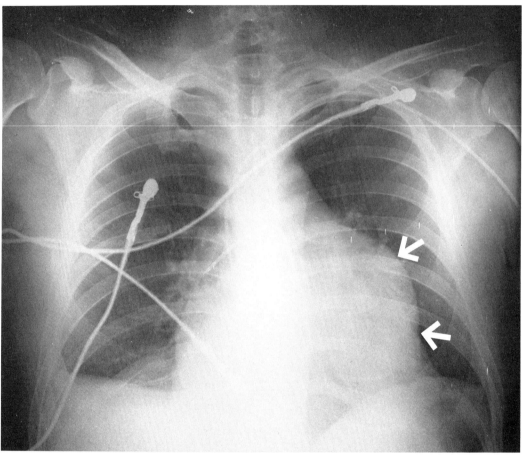

Figure 5–31. Postmitral commissurotomy. *Arrows* demonstrate widened cardiac silhouette from hemopericardium.
   Source: Phillip Cascade, MD.

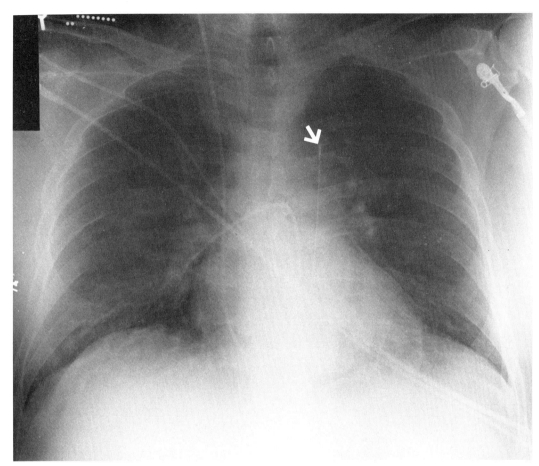

Figure 5–32. Intra-aortic counterpulsation ballon in proper position at aortic arch (*arrow*).
Source: Phillip Cascade, MD.

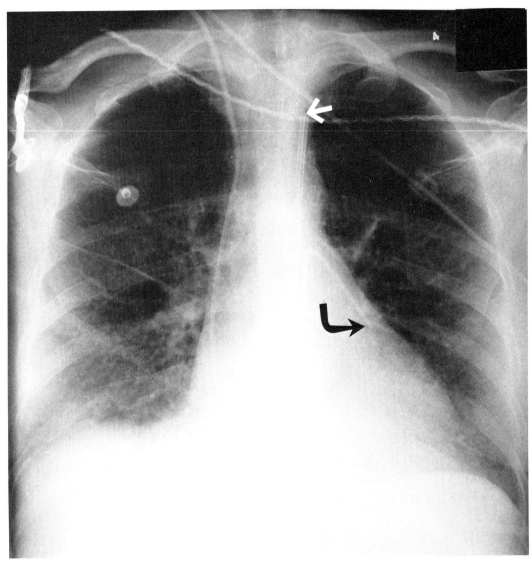

Figure 5–33. Counterpulsation balloon is placed too cephalad in left subclavian artery (*arrow*); Swan-Ganz catheter is placed too distal in left pulmonary artery (*curved arrow*).

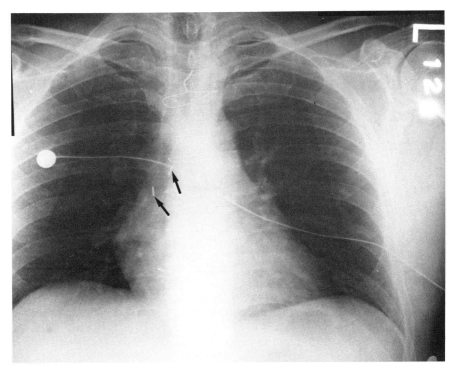

Figure 5–34. Postoperative median sternotomy. **A.** Note markers for bypassed coronary arteries (*arrows*).

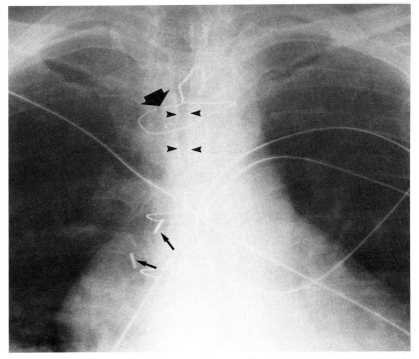

Figure 5–34B. Note sternal dehiscence with separation of bony sternum (*arrowheads*); *large arrow* points to break in circular wire suture, *thin arrows* point to coronary graft markers.

Source: Phillip Cascade, MD

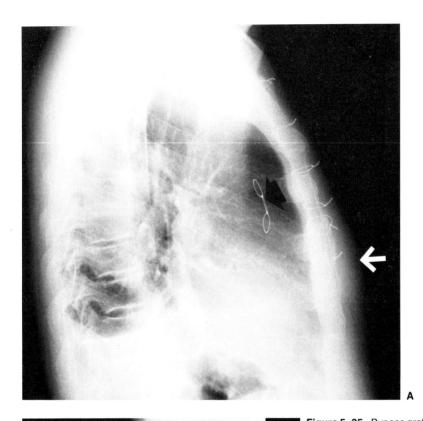

A

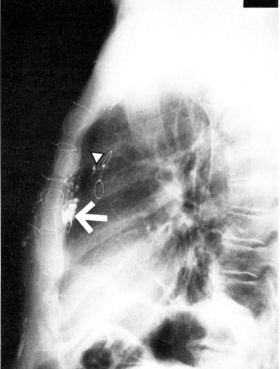

Figure 5–35. Bypass graft markers. **A.** *Large black arrow* demonstrates site of bypass graft; *white arrow* denotes swollen inflamed soft tissues. **B.** Film displays postoperative abscess. *Large arrow* demonstrates contrast material pooling in a retrosternal abscess after injection of the contrast in a cutaneous fistula; *arrowhead* displays contrast tracking to the infected graft site.

Source: Phillip Cascade, MD.

B

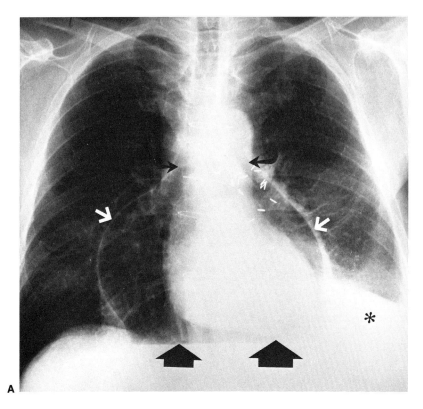

Figure 5–36. Hydropneumopericardium. **A.** Pericardium is displaced by large amount of air (*white arrows*); *large arrows* display air-fluid level; *asterisk* displays left pleural effusion; *curved arrow* displays superior attachment of pericardium on left to main pulmonary artery; *straight black arrow* shows superior extent of air on the right to superior vena cava and ascending aorta. **B.** Lateral view: note margins of hydropericardium on lateral (*large arrows*). Inferior vena cava (*white arrows*) is outlined by pneumopericardium. *Straight thin black arrow* demonstrates superior extent of pneumopericardium on the ascending aorta.

Source: Phillip Cascade, MD.

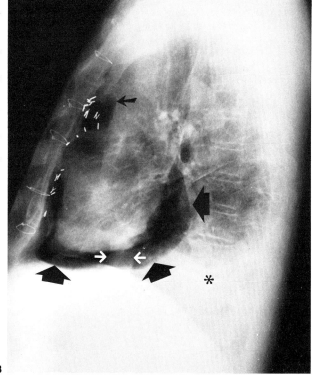

Chapter 6

Catheters and Tubes

Allen J. Stone, MD, *and Lyle D. Victor*, MD

When catheters are inserted for hemodynamic monitoring and central and enteric alimentation, they are frequently malpositioned. The abnormal chest roentgenogram is often the first indicator of complication.

CENTRAL VENOUS PRESSURE CATHETER PLACEMENT

The central venous pressure (CVP) catheter may be used as a conduit for intravenous medications and central hyperalimentation. Most commonly placed by the subclavian or internal jugular route, the tip of the catheter should normally rest between the distal superior vena cava if it is on the "high" side (Fig. 6–1; *wide arrow*) and the right atrium if on the "low" side (Fig. 6–2). An accurate reading can be obtained with the catheter in the innominate vein or in the proximal superior vena, but the more distal location is preferred.

Internal Jugular Site

Malpositioned catheters are too low when they are positioned through the tricuspid valve and rest in the right ventricle (see Fig. 6–15). This displacement can cause valvular damage or can result in ventricular arrhythmias as a result of the catheter striking the ventricular wall. Another low position is shown in Figure 6–3; the

CVP catheter is well below the heart and rests in the inferior vena cava (*black arrow*). Figure 6–4 demonstrates a pulmonary artery catheter introducer being used as a CVP monitor. Spuriously low pressure readings were obtained because the catheter was twisted (*arrow*).

Subclavian Site

Arterial misplacement of CVP catheters can occur in both the internal jugular and subclavian routes of placement. Figure 6–5 shows a CVP catheter placed in the right subclavian artery (*large arrow*) and traversing the innominate artery to rest finally in the aortic knob (*hollow arrow*). Clinical indications that the catheter is in the artery are pulsatile blood return and arterial oxygen tensions measured by arterial blood gases. Unfortunately, in cases of hypotensive, hypoxemic patients these guidelines can be missing. The authors' experience has been that sliding catheters into arteries is more difficult than inserting them into the veins because of the thick elastic properties of the arterial wall. This problem is especially apparent when one is trying to thread a wire introducer in the artery.

Venous malpositions of the catheters are more frequent, however, than arterial malpositions. Figure 6–6 shows a catheter passing from the right subclavian vein to the left subclavian vein and ending in the axillary vein. Figure 6–7A shows a high proximal placement of a right subclavian CVP line (*small arrowhead*). Figure 6–7B shows a subclavian CVP malpositioned in the internal jugular vein.

Catheterization of Pleural Space

Occasionally, a catheter penetrates the subclavian vein and enters the pleural space (Fig. 6–8A). If the malpositioned catheter is not noticed immediately, the rapid collection of pleural fluid will be commensurate with the rate of fluid administration. Figure 6–8B demonstrates opacification of the right hemithorax; it is due to a large pleural infusion. Figure 6–9A shows a left-side catheter that has migrated distally to perforate the innominate vein and to enter the left pleural space, resulting in the development of a pleural effusion (Fig. 6–9B). A short time later the effusion (or infusion in this case) has become massive (Fig. 6–9C). Figure 6–9D shows a Swan-Ganz catheter outlining the internal jugular vein and the oblique left innominate vein. This more angular position of the vein makes easier venous penetration with perpendicularly placed catheters. (Figure 6–8B shows the more commonly seen, less angular, course of the catheter in another patient.)

Broken Catheter

Rarely, during placement of a catheter, the introducing needle can sever the catheter. Figure 6–10 depicts the migration of a broken catheter from the internal jugular vein (Fig. 6–10A) through the right ventricle to the pulmonary artery on the right (Fig. 6–10B).

Local Hematoma

Miscannulation of an artery or venipuncture may result in a local hematoma. Figure 6–11 shows cervical swelling from a hematoma after an internal jugular cannulation attempt on the left side of the neck. The *arrow* on the right side demonstrates a normal skin fold. This fold is lost on the left side because of the large hematoma (*asterisk*).

Thoracic Hematoma

Figure 6–12A demonstrates a CVP catheter (*arrow*) that appears to be proximally placed. However, there was no blood return, and so the catheter was removed. After the catheter was removed, another roentgenogram was obtained (Fig. 6–12B). The second film demonstrates widening of the mediastinum on the right side (*arrows*), due to bleeding in this space. A vascular structure had been perforated by the catheter. The *black arrow* points to the trachea deviated to the left side. Figure 6–12C demonstrates that the hematoma has extended from the mediastinum into the right extrapleural space (*asterisk*). The trachea (*black arrow*) has shifted to the left side because of the massive right-side mediastinal and apical extrapleural hematoma.

PULMONARY ARTERY CATHETER PLACEMENT

Pulmonary artery catheters (Swan–Ganz catheters) are most commonly placed by the internal jugular or subclavian approach. A large-bore, rigid introducing catheter over a previously placed flexible wire is used.

Correctly positioned catheters are maintained just distal to the pulmonary artery outflow tract (Fig. 6–13; see also Fig. 6–7A—(*large arrowhead*). Pulmonary artery catheters can be placed too proximally; for example, in Figure 6–14, the catheter tip is seen in the pulmonary artery outflow tract or the right ventricle. In this patient, a right ventricular pressure tracing was noted, verifying a more proximal placement. Obvious ventricular placement is seen in Figure 6–15. "Proximal" malplacement is seen in Figure 6–16; a subclavian route was used, and the catheter was positioned in the internal jugular vein. Too distal placement of a catheter is shown in Figure 6–17 (also Fig. 6–19A). Both of these catheters demonstrated a wedge tracing on the catheter pressure monitor. Distal positioning may cause a pulmonary infarct like that seen in Figure 6–18 and Figure 6–19A. Figure 6–19B shows a catheter placed too distally in the right upper lobe. In Figures 6–20A and 6–20B, the catheter is positioned in the hepatic vein. The catheter retraced its course after entering the right ventricle (*inferior left arrow*) to pass into the right atrium, the inferior vena cava, and finally wedged into the hepatic vein (*inferior right arrow*). The arrows outline the course of the pulmonary artery catheter from the superior vena cava to the right atrium to the right ventricle, back to the right atrium, and then to the inferior vena cava.

Catheters may coil in the pulmonary artery or right atrium of the heart like that shown in Figure 6–21 (see also Fig. 6–20A). Our experience shows that this complication occurs more often when pulmonary artery or wedge pressures are abnormally high, and thus interfere with adequate distal flow of the inflated balloon.

Catheters can also become knotted (see Fig. 6–19A; *arrowhead*). This situation can lead to a potentially dangerous venous laceration when attempts are made to remove the catheter.

The twisting of introducer sheaths is noticeable on the chest roentgenogram shown in Figure 6–22A (see also Fig. 6–4). A dampened pulmonary artery pressure tracing can occur as a result of partial obstruction of the catheter from the twisting. Figure 6–22B shows a fractured introducing catheter secondary to persistent twisting after a femoral venous insertion.

Figure 6–23 shows a pulmonary artery catheter severed when an attempt was made to change the catheter. The floating ends of the catheter are indicated by the *thin arrows*; the introducer containing the proximal end of the severed catheter, by the *wide arrow*.

NASOGASTRIC AND FEEDING TUBE PLACEMENT

The properly positioned nasogastric tube has the distal tip in the stomach (see Fig. 6–1—*thin arrows*—and Fig. 6–15—*dark wide arrow*). Proximal malpositioning is shown in Figure 6–24 at the level of the midthoracic esophagus (*wide arrows*). Nasogastric tube coiling frequently occurs in intubated patients because of their impaired ability to assist placement by

swallowing and, more importantly, by the obstruction to movement caused by pressure on the esophagus from the inflated cuff of the endotracheal tube. Distal coiling is shown in Figure 6–25. The tube is passing back into the esophagus (*small arrowheads*) and is coiling in a hiatal hernia. For an example of proximal coiling, see Figure 6–5 (*small arrow*).

Feeding tubes differ from nasogastric tubes; they have a mercury tip to encourage gravitational tube positioning in the duodenum and the jejunum. Observation of this opacity on the chest roentgenogram can assist in tube position determinations. Figures 6–26 and 6–27A show the feeding tube in the esophagus. After the patient shown in Figure 6–27 had been placed on her side for three hours, the tip of the feeding tube passed into the jejunum (Fig. 6–27B).

Improperly placed nasogastric and feeding tubes can cause dangerous complications. This possibility is shown in Figure 6–28. The tube was placed in the trachea, migrated to the lateral basal segment of the right lower lobe, and then penetrated the visceral pleura. The result was a pneumothorax (*white arrows*) and a bronchopleural fistula.

Figure 6–29 shows a mercury-tipped feeding tube misplaced in the right mainstem bronchus. In another patient, a mercury bag completely dislodged from the tube and filled the right mainstem bronchus and bronchus intermedius (Fig. 6–30). Because of the risks of tracheal intubation, one must always listen carefully over the epigastrium for gurgling sounds when air is instilled in the newly positioned nasogastric tube.

CHEST TUBE PLACEMENT

Chest tubes may be placed laterally or anteriorly. The properly positioned lateral chest tube shown in Figure 6–31 was placed for removal of a hemopneumothorax after an attempt to insert a subclavian catheter. The *thin arrows* point to the suction side-holes; the *wide arrows* point to the blood layering in the right costophrenic angle; the *white arrow* points to a small residual pneumothorax. A well-positioned lateral chest tube should be no lower than the fifth or sixth intercostal space in order to avoid penetration of the liver or the stomach and the abdominal cavity. The second or third anterior intercostal space in the midclavicular line is the proper entry point for aspiration of a pneumothorax (see Figure 4–2B). As a general rule, the lateral tube position is used to aspirate pleural fluid, and the anterior approach is employed for the aspiration of a pneumothorax. These positions are necessary because fluid layers-out posteriorly in the supine position; whereas, air gravitates anteriorly when the patient is lying on his back.

In Figure 6–32A, too low positioning of the chest tube resulted in gastric insertion (*arrowheads*). A low right-sided insertion is seen in Figure 6–32B. The *blunt arrow* points to the tip abutting the mediastinum. The small-bore chest tube shown in Figure 6–33 was malpositioned in the anterior thoracic wall (*black arrow*). It then passed into the soft tissues (*arrowhead*). Kinking of a chest tube is demonstrated in Figure 6–15.

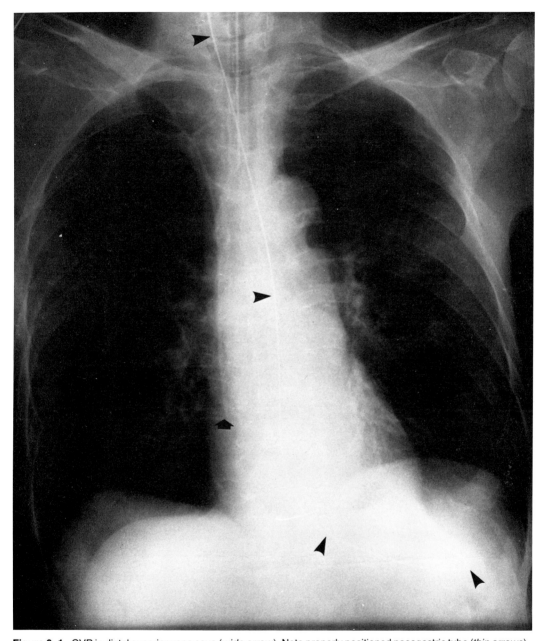

Figure 6–1. CVP in distal superior vena cava (*wide arrow*). Note properly positioned nasogastric tube (*thin arrows*).

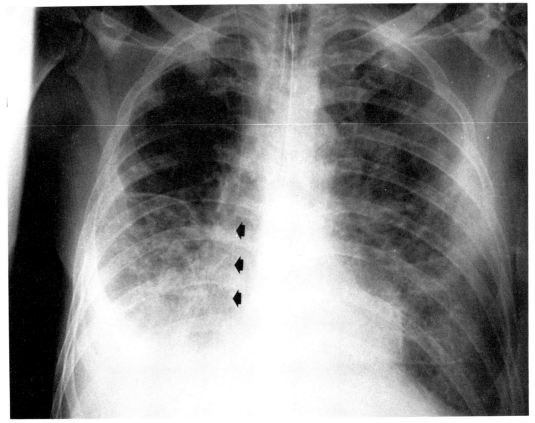

Figure 6–2. CVP in right atrium (*inferior arrow*).

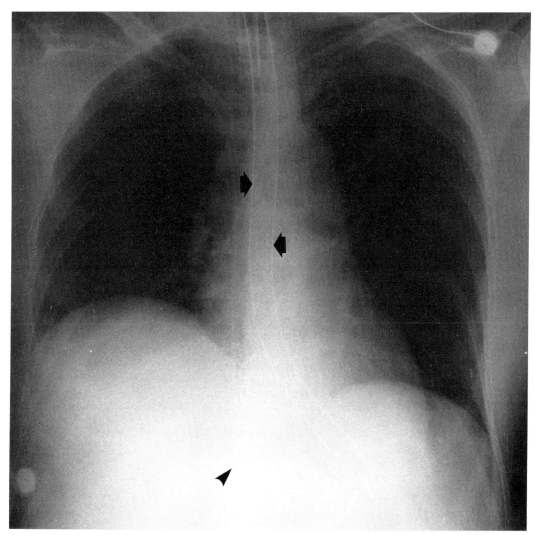

Figure 6–3. CVP on right passing into inferior vena cava (*thin arrow*). Note two NG tubes (*wide arrows*).

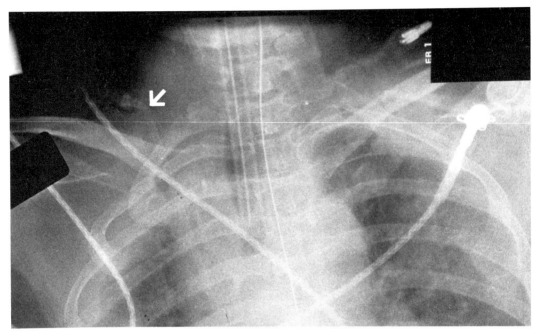

Figure 6–4. Twisted pulmonary artery catheter introducer (*white arrow*).

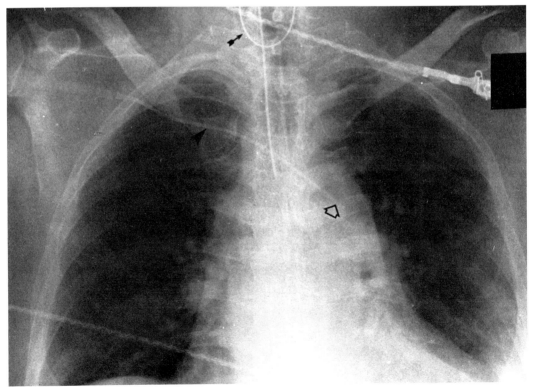

Figure 6–5. Arterial misplacement. CVP catheter is misplaced into right subclavian artery (*wide black arrow*), passes retrograde into the innominate artery, and terminates in the aortic knob (*wide open arrow*). NG tube is coiled in cervical esophagus (*small black arrow*).

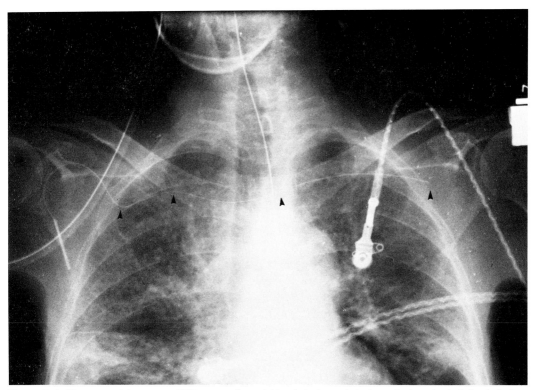

Figure 6–6. Venous malplacement. CVP passes from right subclavian vein to innominate veins to left subclavian vein (*arrowheads*).

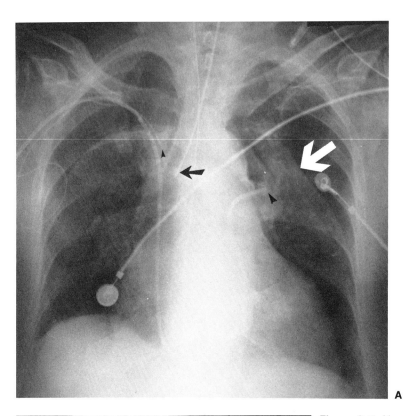

A

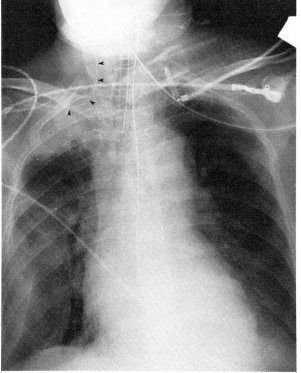

Figure 6–7. Venous malplacement. **A.** Note high placement of CVP on right (*small arrowhead*). Swan-Ganz catheter is in the left pulmonary artery (*large arrowhead*), and endotracheal tube is positioned in the right mainstem bronchus (*black arrow*). Note skin fold (*white arrow*). **B.** CVP passes retrograde from subclavian vein to internal jugular vein (*arrowheads*).

B

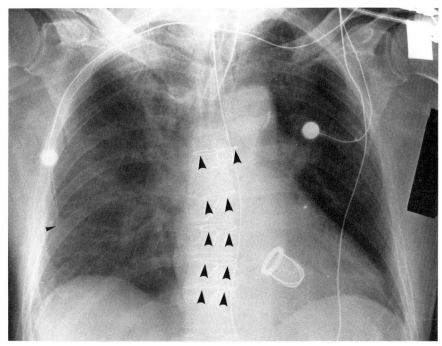

Figure 6–8. Malplaced catheterization of right pleural space. **A.** CVP catheter placed by the internal jugular approach has lodged laterally in the pleural space (*thin arrow*). Note wire sutures in sternum (*wide arrows*); mitral valve prosthesis is located to left of midline in lower left chest.

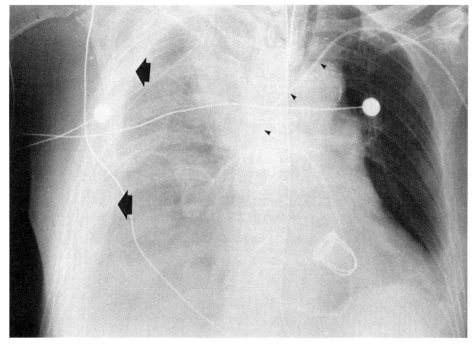

Figure 6–8B. Six hours later, there is general haziness of right hemithorax. It is due to posterior layering of infused Ringer's lactate solution in pleural space. The *wide arrows* point to lateral layering of fluid. Note gentle angular course of left innominate vein with Swan-Ganz catheter in place (*arrowheads*).

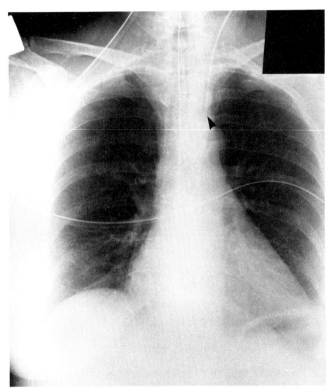

Figure 6–9. Distal migration of catheter to left pleural space. **A.** *Arrow* demonstrates CVP catheter that appears to be in left innominate vein. **B.** Six hours later, catheter has migrated inferiorly below the level of the innominate vein (*arrow*). Note the accumulation of pleural fluid on the left (*asterisk*).

A

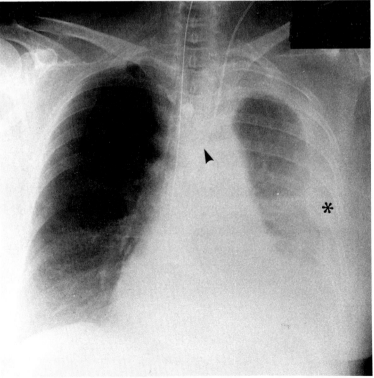

B

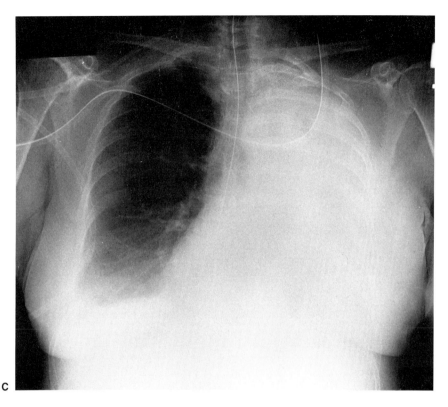

C

Figure 6–9C. Eight hours later, x-ray film shows that catheter has been removed, but entire left hemithorax is opacified because of pleural infusion of Ringer's lactate solution. **D.** *Arrows* demonstrate Swan-Ganz catheter outlining increased angulation of the junction of internal jugular vein and innominate vein.

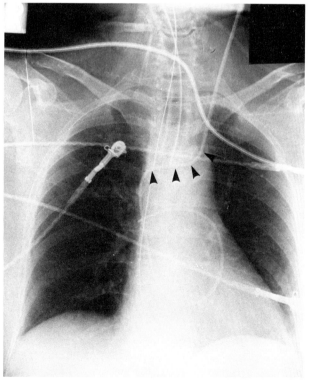

D

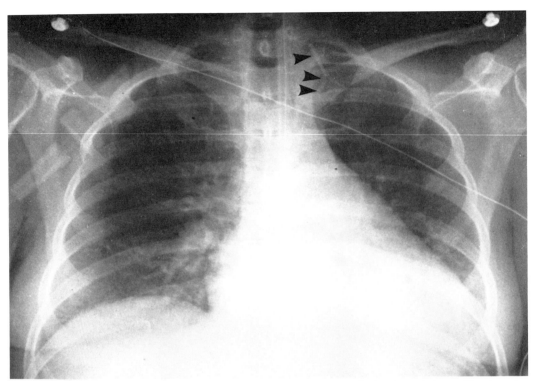

Figure 6–10. Migration of broken catheter. **A.** *Arrows* demonstrate severed CVP catheter in internal jugular vein.

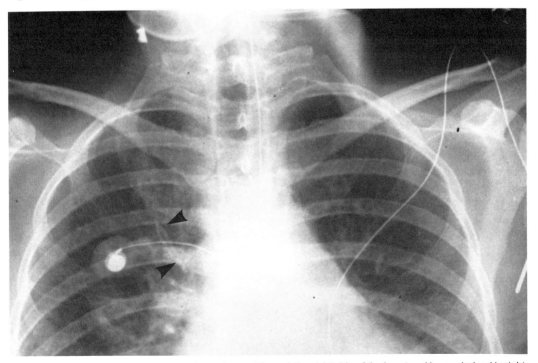

Figure 6–10B. A few days later, catheter has migrated through the right side of the heart and is now lodged in right upper lobe pulmonary artery (*arrows*).

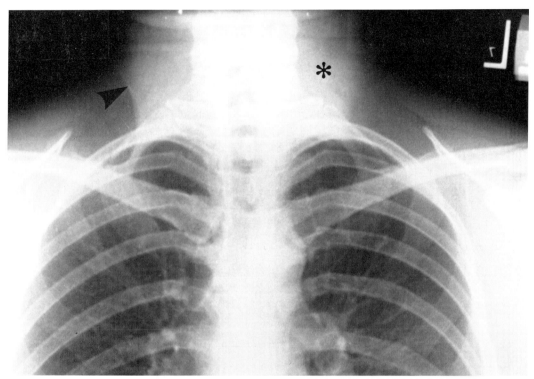

Figure 6–11. Left-side hematoma (*asterisk*) after unsuccessful attempt to insert CVP line in neck. *Large arrow* demonstrates a normal skin fold on the right side that is obscured on the left because of the swelling.

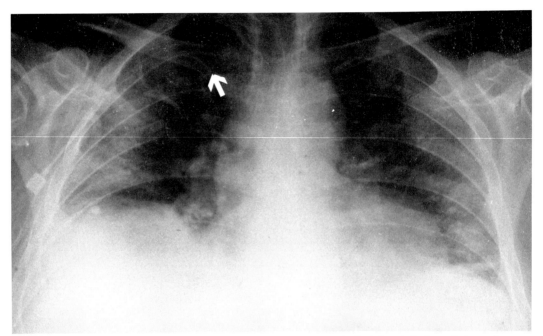

Figure 6–12. Misplaced CVP catheter. **A.** CVP catheter that appears to be in right subclavian vein (*arrow*).

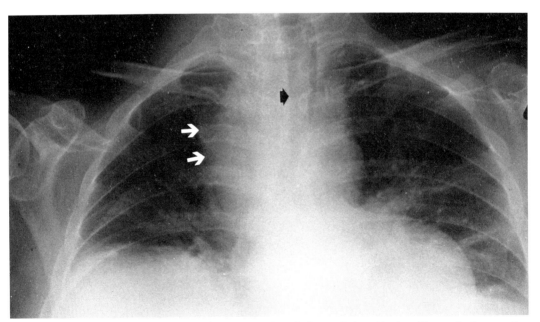

Figure 6–12B. Two hours after catheter has been removed, study demonstrates widening of the mediastinum on the right (*arrows*) because of mediastinal hematoma. Deviation of the trachea to the left (*wide arrow*) is due to mediastinal hematoma.

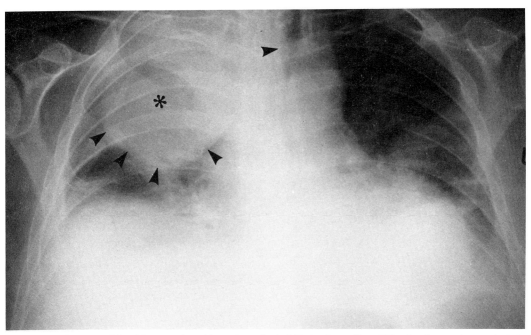

Figure 6–12C. Large right-side extrapleural hematoma (*asterisk*) due to continued bleeding is now demonstrated. This space communicates with the mediastinum. The sharp, smooth margin (*wide arrows*) suggests the extrapleural location. Note persistent tracheal deviation (*arrow*).

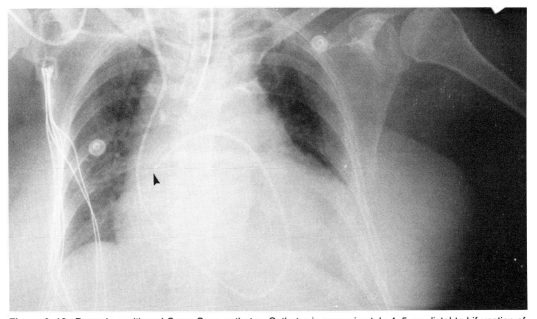

Figure 6–13. Properly positioned Swan-Ganz catheter. Catheter is approximately 4–5 cm distal to bifurcation of pulmonary artery (*arrowhead*).

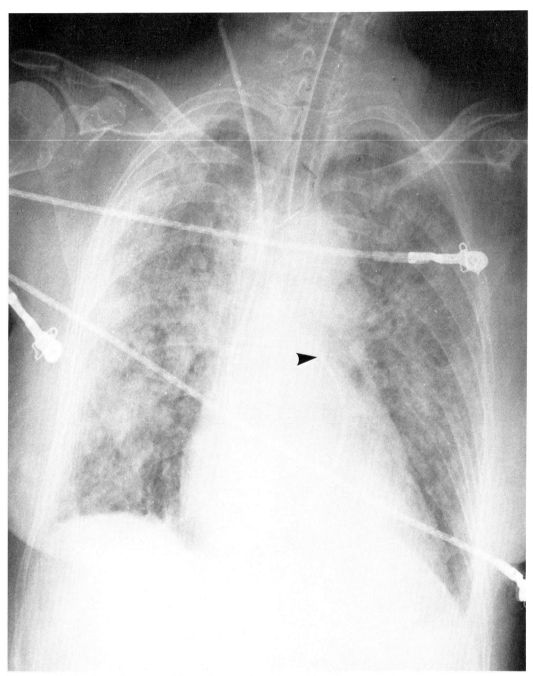

Figure 6–14. Proximal placement of Swan-Ganz catheter (*arrow*) in pulmonary outflow tract. A right ventricular pressure was obtained; patient has cardiogenic pulmonary edema.

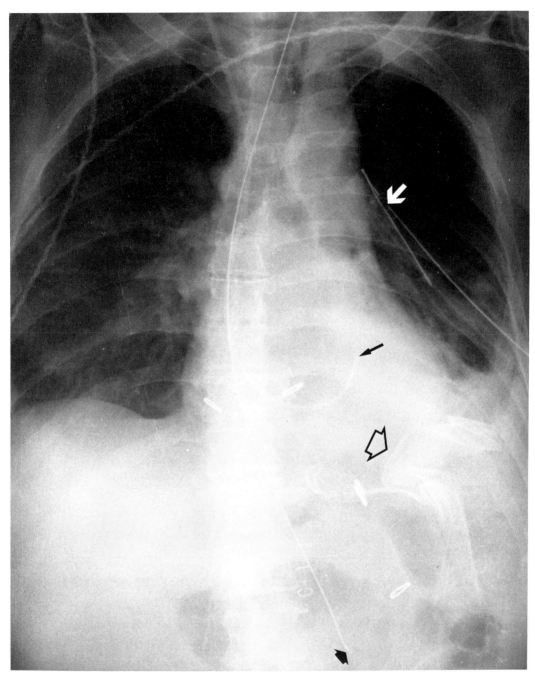

Figure 6–15. Right ventricular placement of Swan-Ganz catheter (*small black arrow*). Thoracotomy tube on left side is kinked on itself (*white arrow*). A Penrose drain (*open arrow*) has been placed beneath the left hemidiaphragm for drainage of subphrenic abscess. Nasogastric tube is properly positioned in stomach (*wide black arrow*).

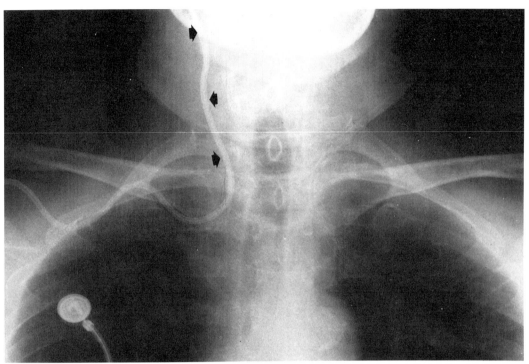

Figure 6–16. Malposition of Swan-Ganz catheter. Passage is in superior direction into internal jugular vein. Note *arrows* pointing to malpositioned catheter.

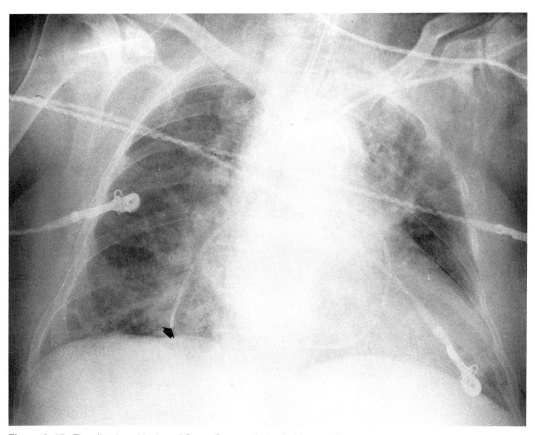

Figure 6–17. Too distal positioning of Swan-Ganz catheter (*wide arrow*).

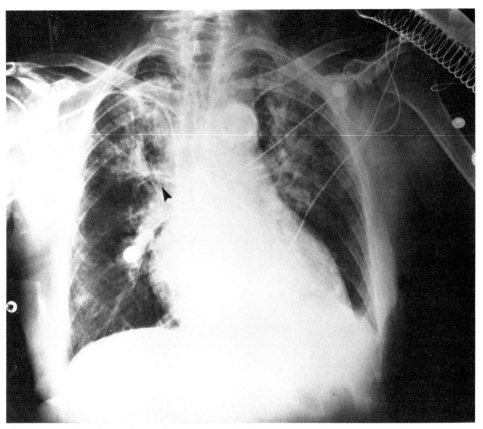

Figure 6–18. *Arrowhead* demonstrates distal end of pulmonary catheter approximating a triangular density that represents a pulmonary infarct.

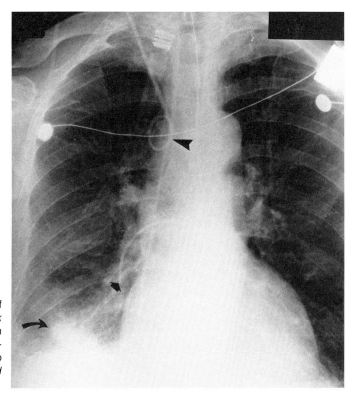

Figure 6-19. Distal placement of Swan-Ganz catheter. **A.** *Wide black arrow* points to Swan-Ganz catheter in peripheral location. This led to pulmonary infarct (*curved arrow*) adjacent to the right hemidiaphragm. *Arrowhead* demonstrates knot in catheter.

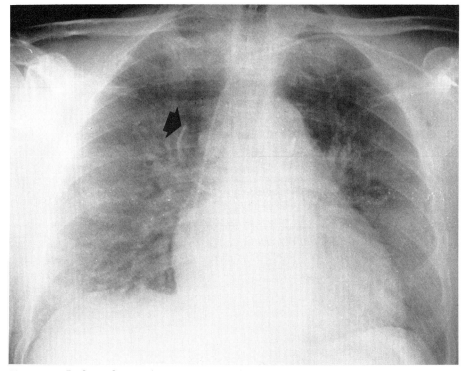

Figure 6-19B. Swan-Ganz catheter malpositioned in right upper lobe (*arrow*).

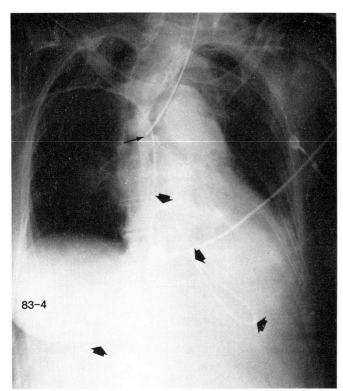

83-4

Figure 6–20 Swan-Ganz catheter mal-placed in hepatic vein. **A.** Film demon-strates a Swan-Ganz catheter that has passed into the right ventricle (*lower left arrow*) and retraced its path into the right atrium (*most superior arrow*), inferior vena cava, and wedged into the hepatic vein (*lower right arrow*). Note endo-tracheal tube passing into right mainstem bronchus (*thin arrow*).

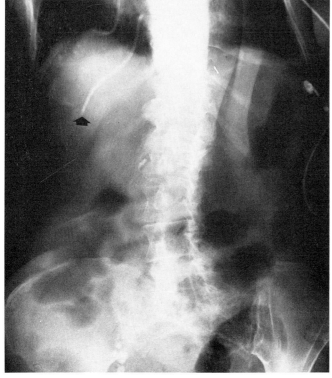

Figure 6–20B. This abdominal film dem-onstrates catheter in hepatic vein (*arrow*).

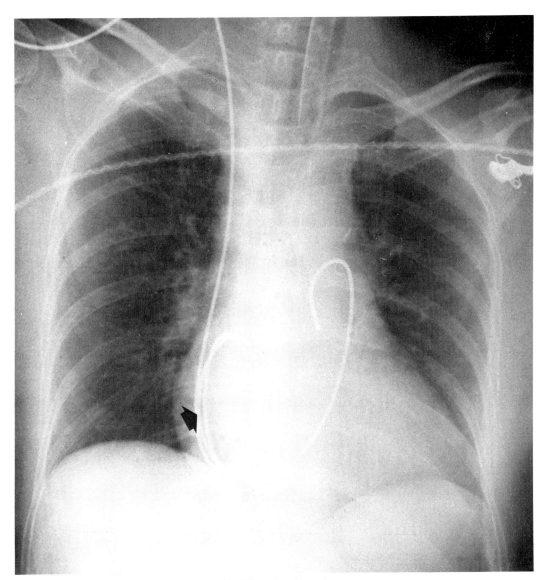

Figure 6–21. Coiled catheter is demonstrated in right atrium (*arrow*).

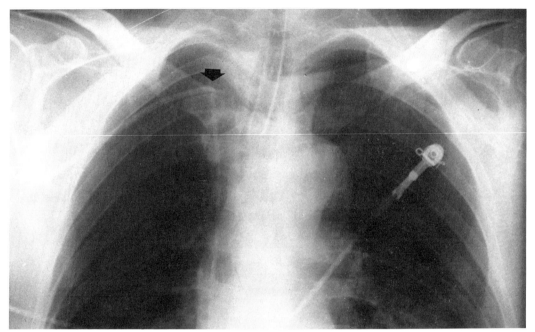

Figure 6–22. Twisting-induced damage to catheters. **A.** Kink in introducing sheath in right subclavian vein (*arrow*).

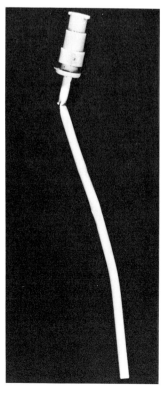

Figure 6–22 B. Introducing catheter fractured secondary to twisting after venous insertion.

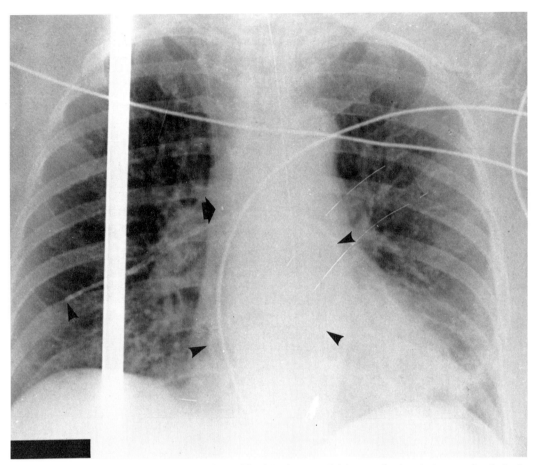

Figure 6–23. Severed pulmonary artery catheter. The introducer containing proximal end of severed catheter is shown by *wide arrow*. Free severed distal catheter is shown by *thin arrows*.

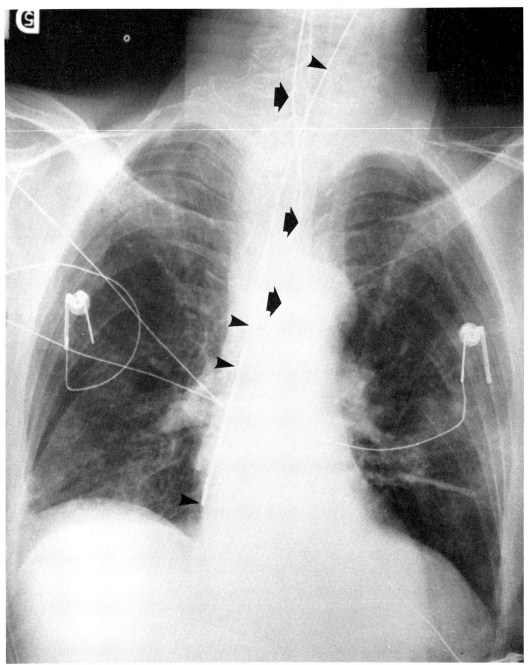

Figure 6–24. Proximal placement of a nasogastric tube in midthoracic esophagus (*wide arrows*). *Thin arrows* demonstrate nasogastric tube outside body.

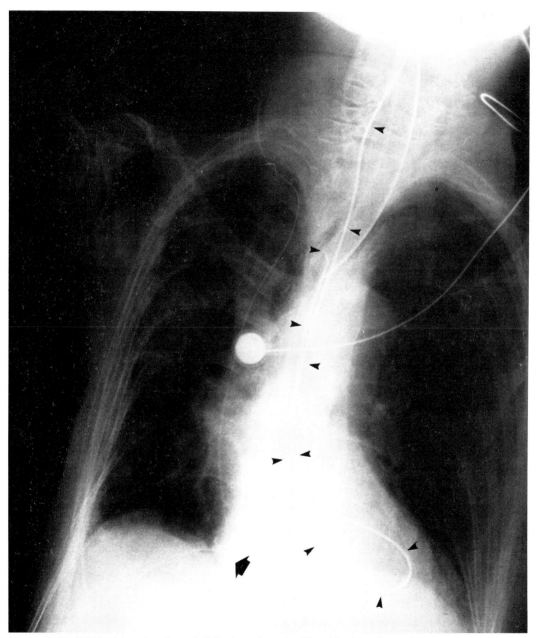

Figure 6–25. CVP in right atrium (*arrow*). NG tube coils on itself in a hiatal hernia passing retrograde in thoracic esophagus (*arrowheads*).

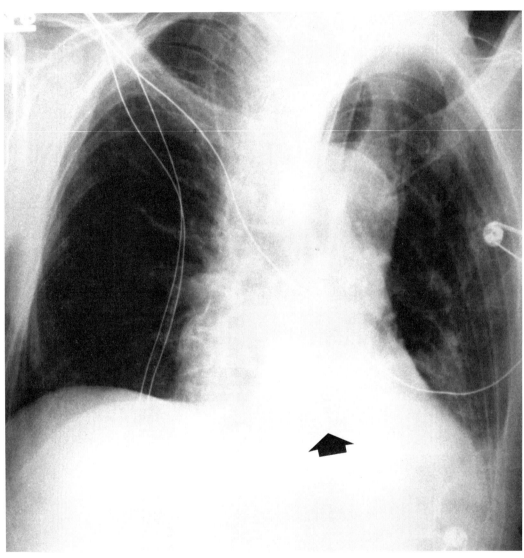

Figure 6–26. Mercury end of feeding tube in distal esophagus (*arrow*).

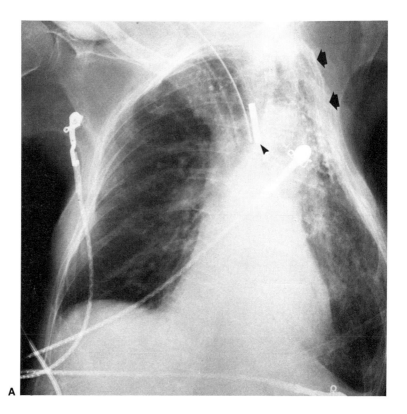

Figure 6–27. Positioning of feeding tube. **A.** Proximal malpositioning of feeding tube (*arrowhead*). Note rib resections of left upper hemithorax, which were performed many years ago to collapse left upper lobe in treatment of pulmonary tuberculosis (*arrows*), known as thoracoplasty. **B.** Feeding tube now in normal position in jejunum (arrow).

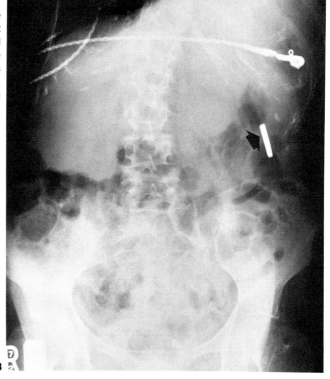

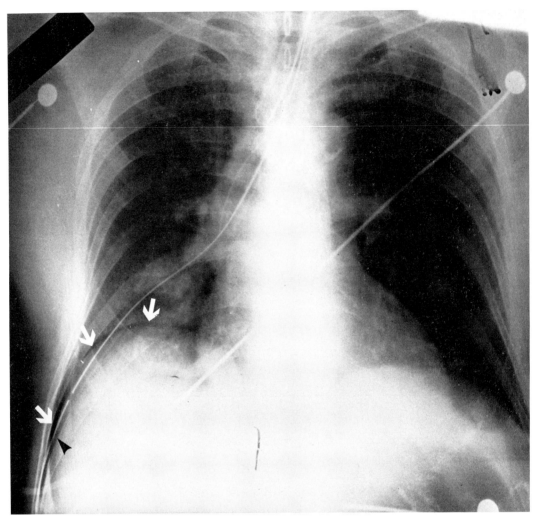

Figure 6–28. Intubation of right lower lobe with nasogastric tube. The tip of feeding tube is seen in costophrenic angle (*arrowhead*). The *white arrows* outline pneumothorax.

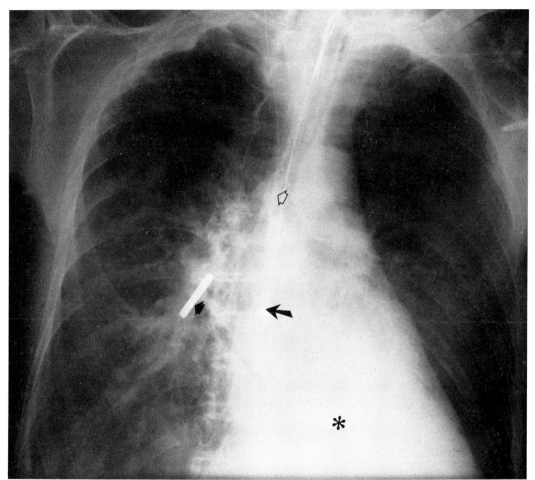

Figure 6–29. Misplaced feeding tube. *Clear arrow* demonstrates feeding tube in trachea passing into right mainstem bronchus; *wide arrow* shows mercury bag in right mainstem bronchus; *large arrow* points to nasogastric tube in the esophagus; atelectasis is demonstrated in the left lower lobe (*asterisk*).

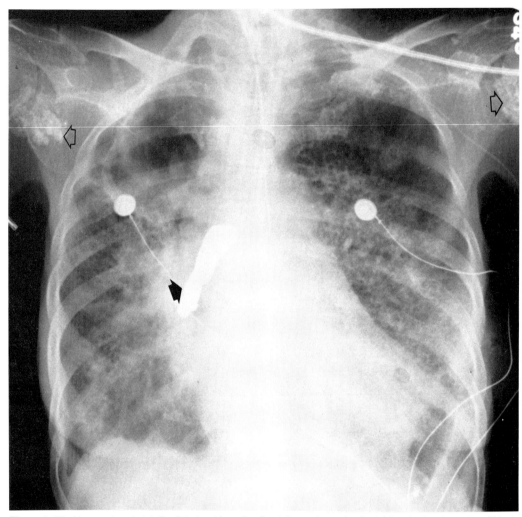

Figure 6–30. Mercury bag is totally dislodged from feeding tube and remains in right mainstem bronchus (*black arrow*). The lungs demonstrate pulmonary edema from renal failure. Note also periarticular calcification in shoulder areas (*open arrows*); it is associated with chronic renal failure.

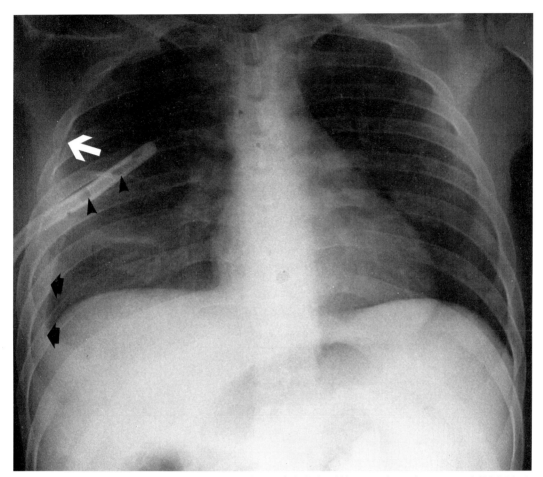

Figure 6–31. Chest tube inserted for hemopneumothorax. Side-holes (*thin arrows*) are demonstrated. *Thick black arrows* demonstrate pleural fluid layering laterally. *White arrow* demonstrates visceral pleural line with pneumothorax lateral to it.

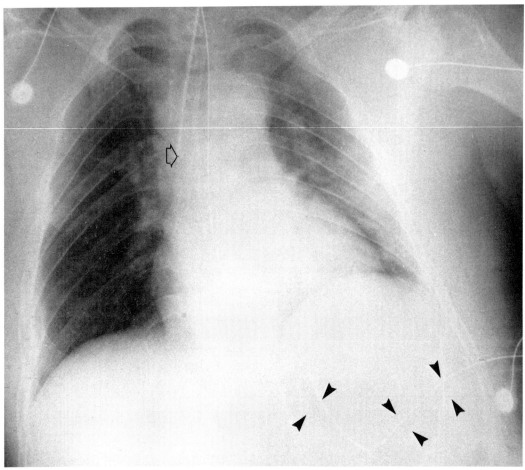

Figure 6–32A. Malpositioned chest tube. **A.** *Black arrowheads* identify chest tube malpositioned below left hemidiaphragm with gastric insertion. Endotracheal tube is positioned in right mainstem bronchus and causes decreased aeration of left lung (*open arrow*).

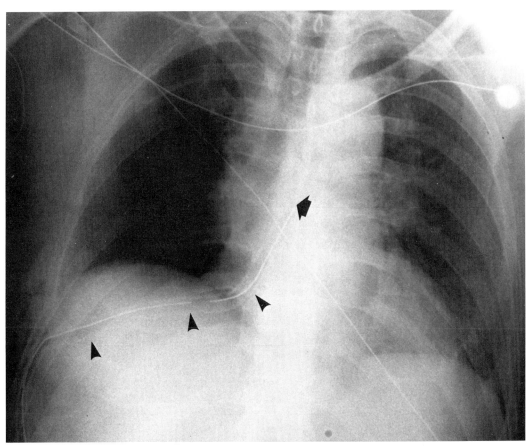

Figure 6–32B. Note low lateral positioning of right sided chest tube (*thin arrows*). Distal tip abuts on mediastinum.

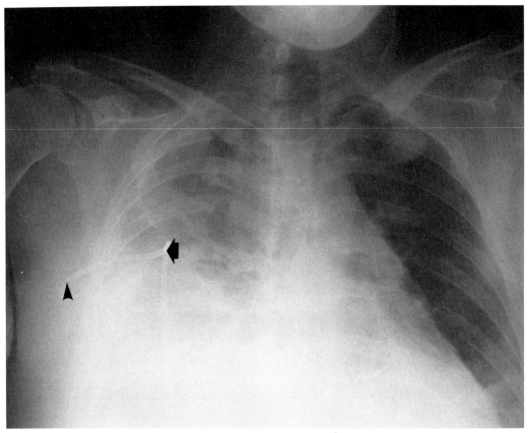

Figure 6–33. Chest tube inserted for pleural effusion. *Arrow* points to site of insertion. The tube passed into soft tissues in a lateral direction without penetrating pleural space (*arrowhead*).

Chapter 7

Complications of Intubation and Tracheostomy*

Lyle D. Victor, MD, *Allen J. Stone*, MD, *and Thomas A. Kwyer*, MD

ENDOTRACHEAL INTUBATION

Proper positioning of the endotracheal tube is important because it ensures adequate pulmonary toilet and mechanical ventilation. Unfortunately, the most commonly seen tracheal complications in the intensive care unit are those secondary to endotracheal intubation. Roentgenography can assist hospital personnel in making proper placement of endotracheal and tracheal tubes. However, an understanding of normal anatomical relationships is necessary in order to formulate an accurate roentgenographic interpretation of the proper endotracheal tube position.

The relationship of the bifurcation of the trachea (carina) to the endotracheal tube must be established on the chest roentgenogram. However, if the carina cannot be clearly visualized on the x-ray film, an approximation of its location can be made by counting the dorsal vertebrae. On the portable chest roentgenogram the carina is located between vertebrae T-5 and T-7 in 95% of patients.[1] There are 12 thoracic vertebrae, which articulate with the ribs. If the ribs are counted from above (see Fig. 7–1A), the corresponding vertebral body can be found by moving medially. There are also 7 cervical vertebrae, and these can be counted from the thoracic vertebrae (in reverse order) or from the skull. The proper position of the distal end of the endo-

tracheal tube is 5 to 7 cm above the carina, allowing for a 2-cm migration inferiorly when the head is flexed from neutral and a 2-cm ascent when the head is extended. With the head in a neutral position, the endotracheal tube can be placed at the T-3 or the T-4 location for adequate position. The radiograph can demonstrate the head in neutral position if the mandible is superimposed over the C-6 vertebra. With the head in extension, the mandible can be seen over the C-4 vertebra or above (Fig. 7–1B; *white arrow*). Also with the head in extension, the endotracheal tube should not be more than 9 cm above the carina, because in that case the cuff of the tube will be in the larynx. In flexion, the mandible is over the upper dorsal spine, and so the endotracheal tube should be at least 1 cm above the carina.

Endotracheal tubes that are positioned properly may appear to be malpositioned when the patient's head is rotated. For example, Figure 7–1C shows that the endotracheal tube is positioned on the left. This positioning has occurred because the patient has rotated his head and neck to the left posterior oblique position. Figure 7–1D demonstrates that turning the head and neck to a right posterior oblique position causes the tube to be positioned to the right.

The most common complication of endotracheal intubation is malpositioning of the tube in the right mainstem bronchus (Fig. 7–2). Because of the straight take-off of the right mainstem bronchus, the endotracheal tube—if

---

*Cadaver photographs with the assistance of Thomas Kwyer, M.D.

pushed too far distally—invariably lodges on the right side. This placement results in excessive ventilation of the right lung, accompanied by hypoventilation and atelectasis of the left lung. Inasmuch as the total mechanical ventilatory tidal volume may enter the right side, reduced breath sounds are heard on the left side or in the right upper lobe area if its orifice has been passed by the tip of the endotracheal tube. Excessive ventilatory pressures may be required because of decreased compliance from right lung hyperexpansion or from collapse from barotrauma induced pneumothorax. Figure 7–3A shows another right mainstem bronchus intubation—this time, with additional atelectasis of the right upper lobe because the tip of the endotracheal tube has been pushed past the take-off of the right upper lobe bronchus. Atelectasis of the left lung is also present on the roentgenogram. Auscultation of the anterior chest in this patient revealed absent breath sounds on the left and decreased breath sounds in the right upper lobe area. Figure 7–3B was taken after partial withdrawal of the endotracheal tube above the carina (*arrow*). Both upper lobes are not expanded, and the hyperinflation of the right lower lobe is reduced.

Figure 7–4 provides an example of an endotracheal tube positioned too high at the level of the true cords (*thin arrow*). The mandible is obviously above the C-4 vertebral level, indicating that the head is hyperextended. The hyperextension caused the tube to ascend to this dangerous level.

The high placement of the endotracheal tube shown in Figure 7–4 also places the balloon cuff proximal to the vocal cords; this placement leaves the lungs unprotected. Some ventilation could be effected, but aspiration of gastric contents also easily occurred, accounting for the diffuse infiltrates seen in this chest roentgenogram.

ESOPHAGEAL INTUBATION

Malpositioning of the endotracheal tube can occur because of the patulous orifice of the esophagus and its close proximity to the larynx, just posterior and lateral to it. Figures 7–5A and 7–5B show esophageal intubation with a balloon cuffed endotracheal tube on an anterior-posterior (AP) roentgenogram. The tube is laterally placed in relation to the midline trachea (*small arrows*). This abnormal placement is seen on the lateral view of Figure 7–5B, which shows the tube in the esophagus (*arrowheads*) and posterior to the trachea (*curved arrowheads*). Figures 7–6A through 7–6C show a patient in whom the esophagus was perforated during an intubation attempt. Massive amounts of air enter the mediastinum and follow tissue planes into the neck and the anterior chest (7–6A; *white arrows*). An esophagram (Fig. 7–6B) verified the perforation. The presence of barium outside the esophagus and in the neck (*black arrow*) demonstrates a localized perforation of the esophagus. There is increased prevertebral space with air present in it; the esophagus is deviated anteriorly. Perforation of the tissues just lateral to the larynx can occur during a difficult intubation like that shown in Figure 7–7. Figure 7–7A shows the tip of the endotracheal tube in the pyriform sinus, just lateral to the larynx. Figure 7–7B shows the tube positioned in the mediastinum subsequent to intentional perforation.

COMPLICATIONS OF TRACHEOSTOMY

Figures 7–8A and 7–8B show a normally positioned tracheostomy tube in place. Note the midline position of the tracheostomy tube with its distal tip well above the carina (Fig. 7–8A). The ideal position of the distal end of the tracheostomy tube is midway between the stoma (*large arrow*) and the carina (*small arrow*). Figure 7–9 shows an eccentrically placed tube, the placement of which resulted in partial obstruction because its lumen abutted the tracheal wall. The increasing of pressure was required in order to maintain an adequate tidal volume while this patient was on the mechanical ventilator. Overinflation of the balloon in another patient (Fig. 7–10) caused distal obstruction by engulfing the distal end of the tube.

A frequently fatal complication of tracheostomy malposition is paratracheal intubation (Fig. 7–11). Occasionally, a tracheostomy is accidentally dislodged from the tracheal stoma. When reinsertion into the tracheal orifice is attempted, the tracheal lumen is bypassed as the tube travels caudally through the planes of the mediastinum. This cadaver reconstruction demonstrates how the malposition might appear on a chest roentgenogram. Massive subcutaneous and mediastinal emphysema would occur in this situation—especially when mechanical ventilation is attempted.

Tracheomalacia, a pathologic dilatation of the tracheal wall, is seen most often in patients with prolonged endotracheal or tracheostomy tube intubation. There is a weakening of the tracheal wall, due usually to pressure necrosis of the cartilaginous endotracheal rings from the dilated balloon of the tube cuff. Infection may also cause destruction of the cartilaginous rings. Figure 7–12 is a chest roentgenogram of a patient who had a tracheostomy for over two years. Note the dilatation of the tracheal wall at the point where the balloon is inflated (*large arrows*) when compared with the more proximal trachea (*small arrows*).

Tracheal stenosis is another complication of prolonged endotracheal tube-cuff inflation. Figures 7–13A and 7–13B demonstrate tracheal stenosis at the site of previous cuff inflation. The increased cuff pressure overcomes the capillary pressure to the mucous membrane and causes necrosis with eventual stenosis. The cuff should not dilate the trachea more than 1½ times its normal diameter.[1]

OTHER TRACHEAL-ESOPHAGEAL DISORDERS

Foreign bodies in the tracheobronchial tree are frequently seen in children. Figures 7–14A and 7–14B are chest roentgenograms of a child who aspirated a spring from a ball-point pen. Note the spring's location in the right mainstem bronchus. If a foreign body lodges in a bronchus, air can be trapped during respiration. Figures 7–15A through 7–15C demonstrate unilateral inspiratory and expiratory emphysema; tomography displays a foreign body in the right mainstem bronchus. Children with these problems can also have atelectasis. In some cases it is possible to demonstrate a shift of the mediastinum on inspiration toward the affected side and then a shift away from the abnormal side on expiration. Figures 7–16A and 7–16B demonstrate a coin lodged in the proximal thoracic esophagus.

Tracheal deviation can also occur from mediastinal masses. Such a mass is shown in the films of a patient with a substernal thyroid that displaces the trachea to the right (Fig. 7–17A) and anteriorly (Fig. 7–17B).

LARYNGEAL DISORDERS: UPPER AIRWAY OBSTRUCTION

Acute epiglottitis is a common cause of acute upper airway obstruction in children and in adolescents. Often preceded by an upper respiratory tract infection and accompanied by severe sore throat, it rapidly progresses to upper airway obstruction from the hyperemic, swollen epiglottis. If a child has high fever, dyspnea, drooling, and sternal retractions, a lateral soft-tissue roentgenogram of the neck should be performed. Figure 7–18A shows an enlarged, swollen epiglottis in a 14-year-old youth. Forty-eight hours later, the roentgenogram shown in Figure 7–18B was taken; it shows an almost normal epiglottis. Figure 7–19 shows an almost totally obstructed trachea in a case of acute epiglottitis. Swollen tonsils also can cause upper airway obstruction (Fig. 7–20). This young patient developed sleep apnea in the supine position because of positional obstruction to the upper trachea.

NOTE

1. Goodman L, Putnam CE: *Intensive Care Radiology: Imaging of the Critically Ill.* Philadelphia, WB Saunders Co., 1983, pp 18–41.

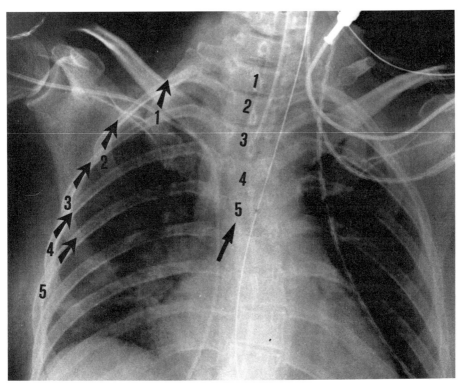

Figure 7–1. Determination of the proper position of the endotracheal tube. **A.** The location of the carina between T-5 and T-7 thoracic vertebrae is found by first counting posterior ribs laterally and then moving medially to locate the corresponding vertebra. Cervical vertebrae can be counted in a reverse fashion from the first thoracic vertebra. Lateral arrows point to rib margins. Medial arrow points to the carina.

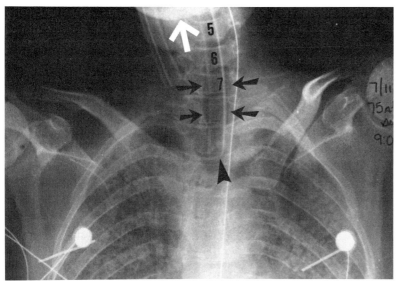

Figure 7–1B. Head in extension. The mandible is seen over the C-4 vertebra (*white arrow*). Lateral margins of the endotracheal tube are shown by *arrows*. The tip of the endotracheal tube in this case is about 7 cm. above the carina.

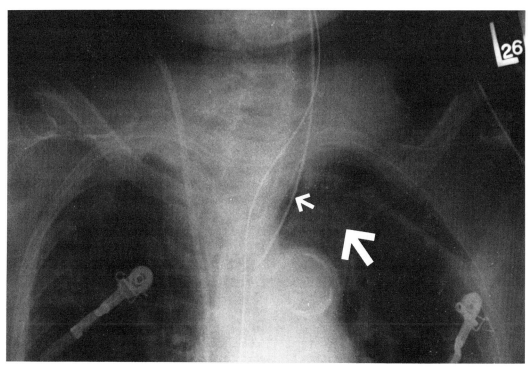

Figure 7–1C. Left neck rotation. Properly positioned endotracheal tube appears to be on the left because of oblique positioning (*small arrow*). Large white arrow shows left clavicle foreshortened verifying oblique position of patient.

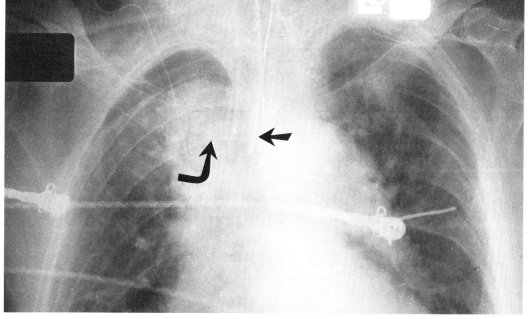

Figure 7–1D. Right neck rotation. Properly positioned endotracheal tube appears to be on right because of oblique positioning (*small arrow*). Curved arrow points to foreshortened right clavicle verifying rotated positioning.

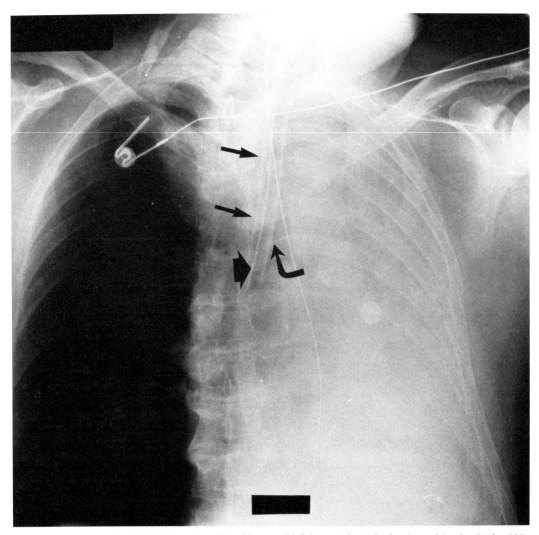

Figure 7–2. Endotracheal intubation malposition. Note total left lung atelectasis due to endotracheal tube (*thin arrows*) obstructing left mainstem bronchus (*curved arrow*). Distal end of the tube is in right mainstem bronchus (*wide arrow*); there is hyperinflation on the right side.

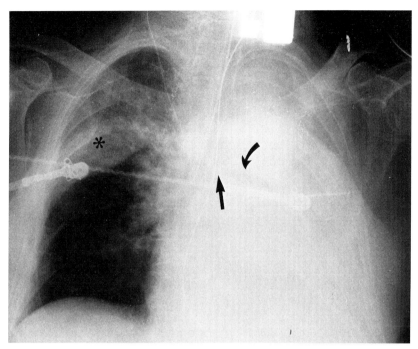

Figure 7–3. Right mainstem bronchus intubation. **A.** Endotracheal tube positioned in right bronchus intermedius is obstructing left main bronchus (*curved arrow*) and causing a left lung atelectasis. It is also obstructing the right upper lobe bronchus and is causing right upper lobe atelectasis (*asterisk*). *Straight arrow* denotes the carina.

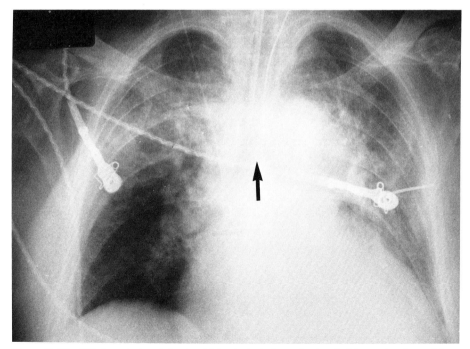

Figure 7–3B. Withdrawal of endotracheal tube to just above the level of the carina (*arrow*) has allowed increased aeration of left lung and right upper lobe. The *straight arrow* denotes the carina.

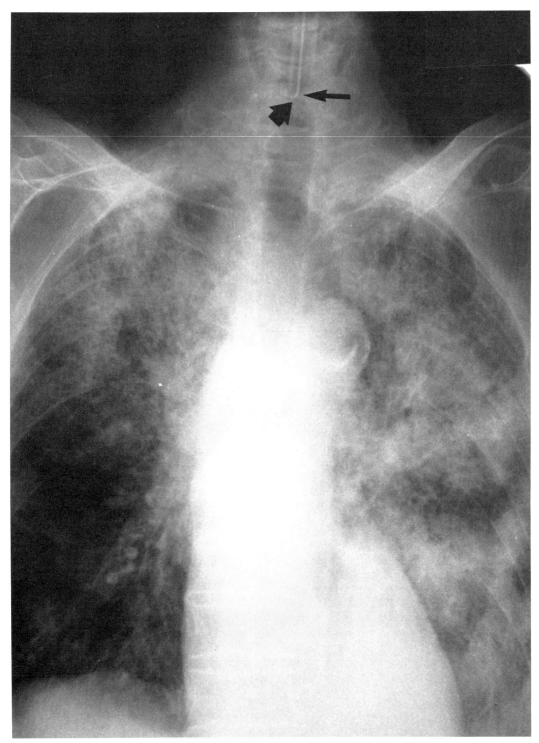

Figure 7–4. High position of endotracheal tube (*wide arrow*) at level of true cords of larynx (*thin arrow*). Mandible is above level of C-4, indicating hyperextension of the neck and allowing endotracheal tube to ascend into larynx. Note bilateral infiltrates of aspiration pneumonitis.

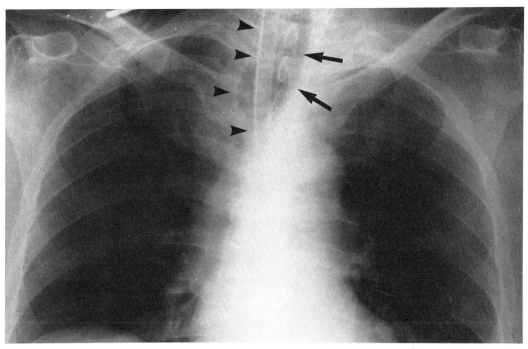

Figure 7–5. AP view of esophageal intubation (*arrowheads*). **A.** The cuff is dilated; note midline position of trachea (*arrows*).

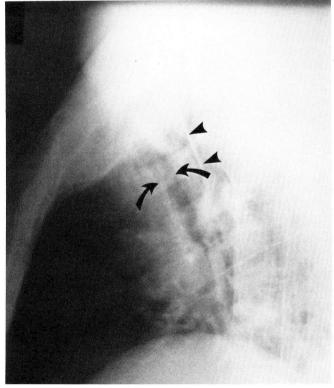

Figure 7–5B. Lateral view displays posterior position of endotracheal tube in esophagus (*arrowheads*). Trachea is located anteriorly (*curved arrows*).

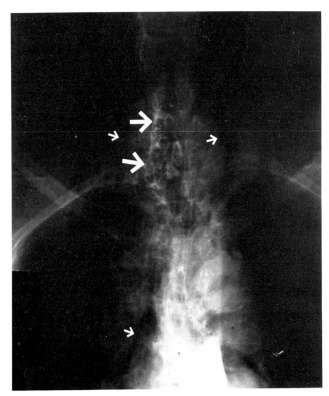

Figure 7–6. Perforation of esophagus. **A.** Note subcutaneous air in neck and mediastinum (*small white arrows*); also note barium extravasated into soft tissues of neck (*large white arrows*).

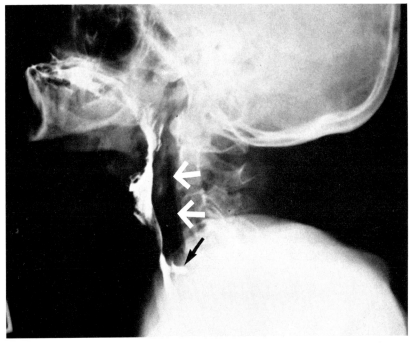

Figure 7–6B. Esophagram demonstrates posterior perforation (*black arrow*). Esophagus is displaced anteriorly by abscess containing air in the prevertebral space (*white arrows*).

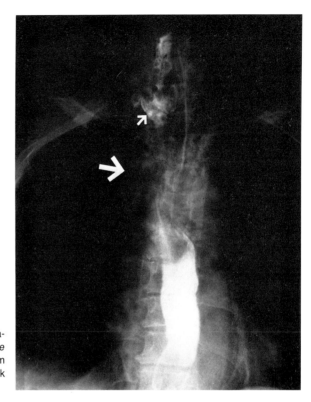

Figure 7–6C. Frontal or AP view displays extravasated barium in neck (*small white arrow*); *large white arrow* demonstrates mediastinal air from perforated esophagus; fascial planes of the neck communicate with the mediastinal spaces.

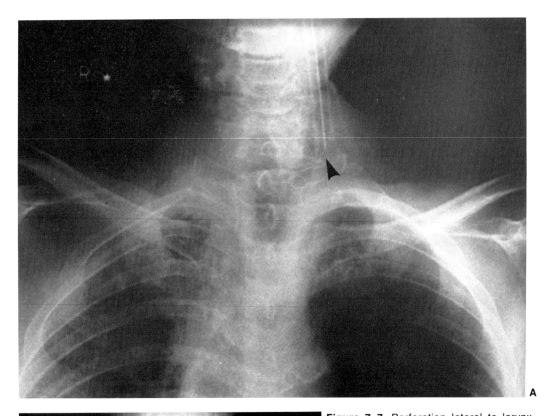

A

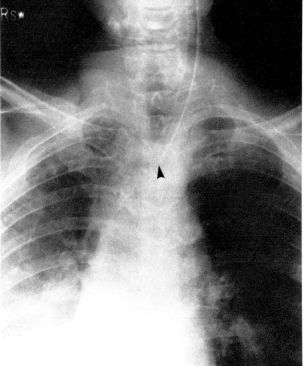

B

Figure 7–7. Perforation lateral to larynx. **A.** Endotracheal tube malpositioned in a cadaver is in left pyriform sinus (arrowhead). **B.** Pyriform sinus has been perforated by endotracheal tube, which is now in mediastinum (*black arrowhead*).

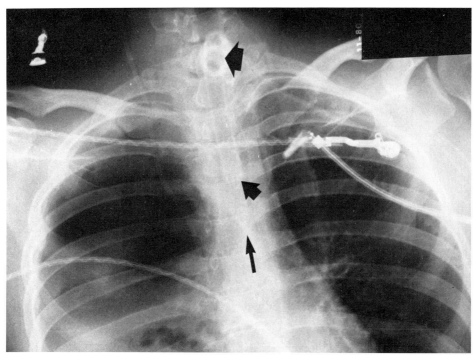

Figure 7–8. Tracheostomy tube in proper position. **A.** Note stoma (*large blunt arrow*), distal end of tracheostomy tube (*small blunt arrow*), and carina (*thin arrow*).

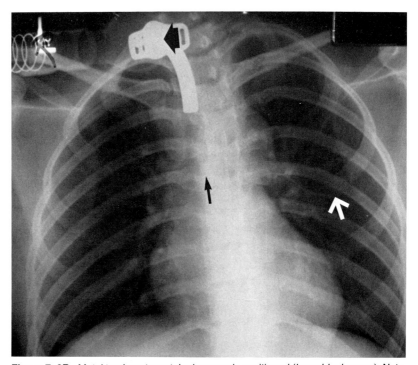

Figure 7–8B. Metal tracheostomy tube is properly positioned (*large black arrow*). Note carina (*thin arrow*) and severed catheter floating freely in pulmonary artery (*white arrow*).

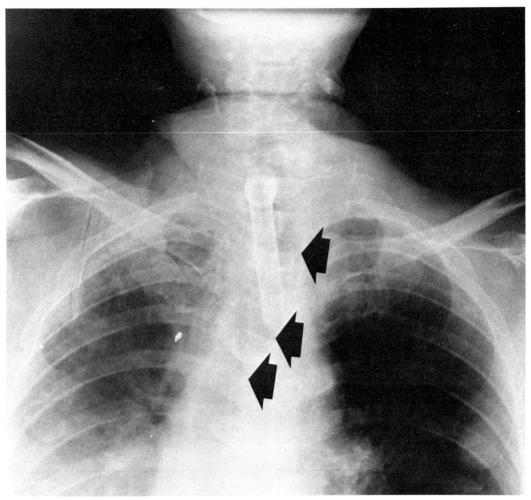

Figure 7–9. Eccentrically placed tracheostomy tube. Malplacement can cause obstruction or erosion of tracheal wall. *Arrows* demonstrate left wall of trachea.

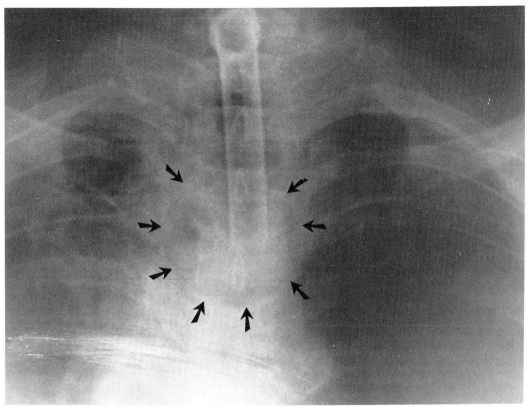

Figure 7–10. Overinflated balloon cuff. Marked overinflation (*arrows*) extends distally and obstructs tracheostomy tube.

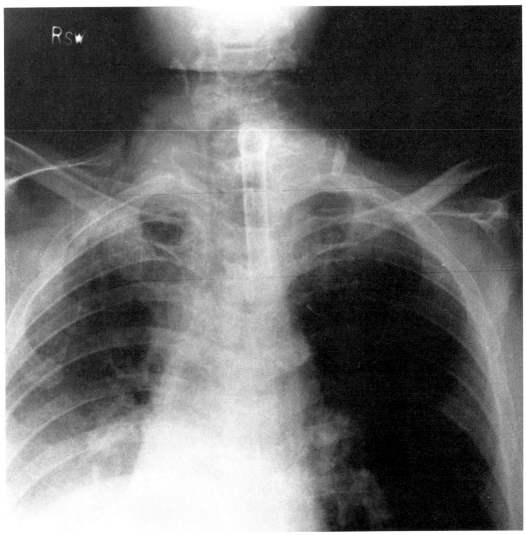

Figure 7–11. Paratracheal intubation of a tracheostomy tube in a cadaver. Tube is located in subcutaneous tissues lateral to trachea.

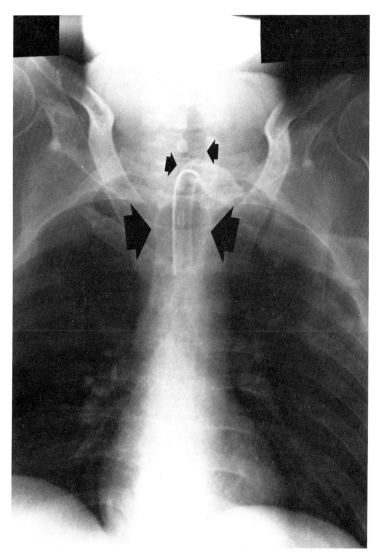

Figure 7–12. Tracheomalacia. Note normal diameter of trachea (*small arrows*); *large arrows* demonstrate dilatation of trachea from tracheomalacia caused by prolonged and excessive cuff dilatation.

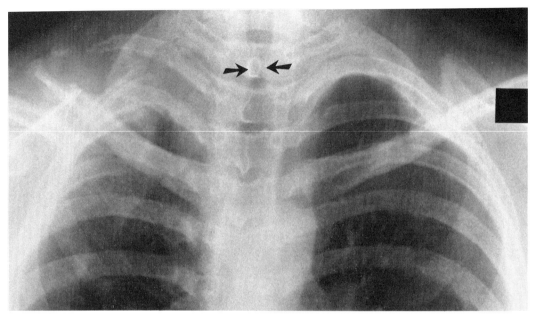

Figure 7–13. Tracheal stenosis. **A.** *Arrows* demonstrate localized area of tracheal stenosis.

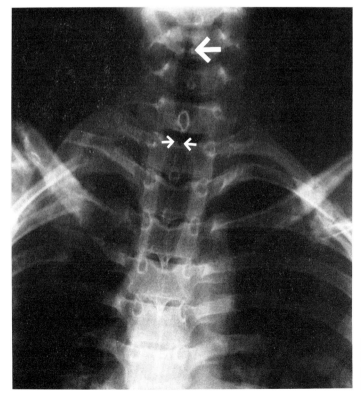

Figure 7–13B. *Small white arrows* indicate tracheal stenosis. Proximal area of narrowing represents normal larynx (*large arrow*).

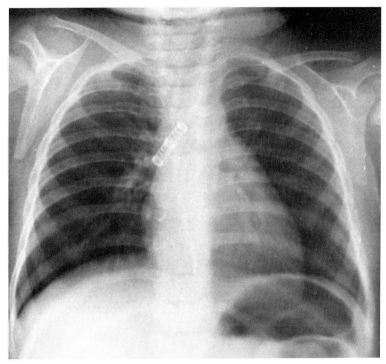

Figure 7–14. Foreign body in tracheobronchial tree. **A.** PA view of aspirated spring from ball-point pen in the right mainstem bronchus.

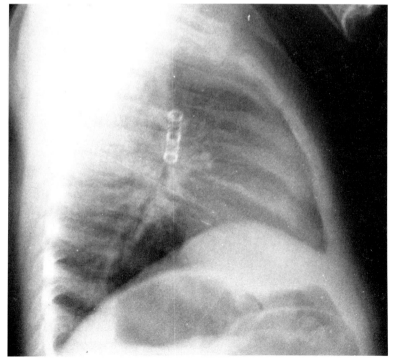

Figure 7–14B. Lateral view.

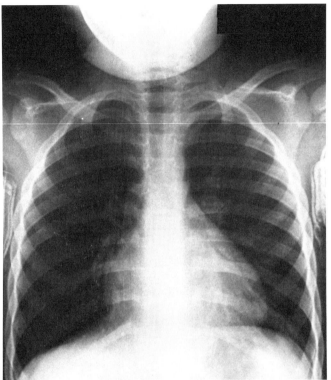

Figure 7–15. Aspiration of a peanut in right mainstem bronchus. **A.** On inspiration both lungs appear well-aerated with greater inflation on right side. **B.** On expiration, there is greater degree of density in left lung because of normal deflation; however, on right side there is obstruction to egress of air, with evidence of obstructive emphysema.

A

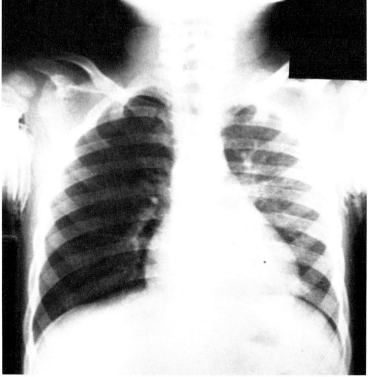

B

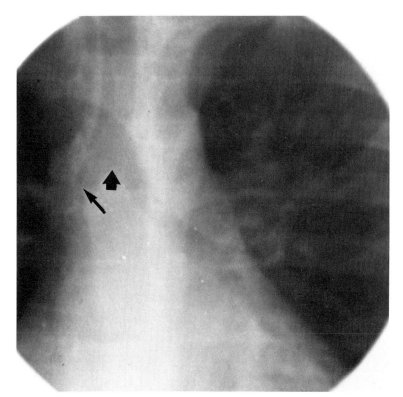

Figure 7–15C. Closeup of tomogram (same patient) demonstrates carina (*wide arrow*); *narrow arrow* is superimposed over foreign body in right mainstem bronchus.

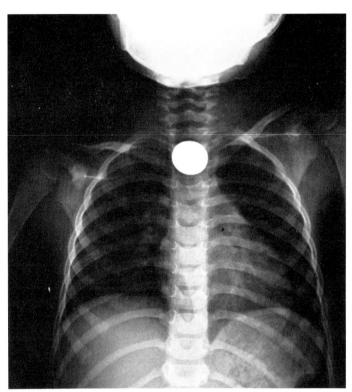

Figure 7–16. Foreign body in esophagus. **A.** PA chest roentgenogram demonstrates coin in the proximal thoracic esophagus.

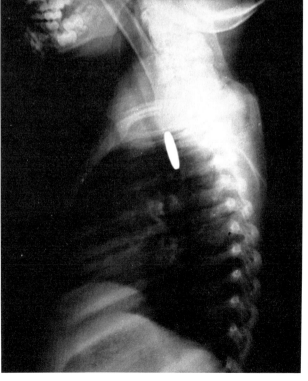

Figure 7–16B. Lateral view.

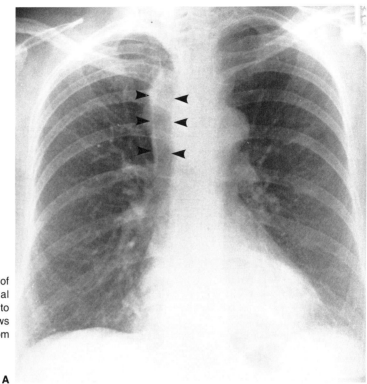

Figure 7–17. Deviation as result of mediastinal mass. **A.** Substernal thyroid mass displaces trachea far to right (*arrowheads*). **B.** Mass bows trachea forward (*arrowheads*) from its posterior location.

A

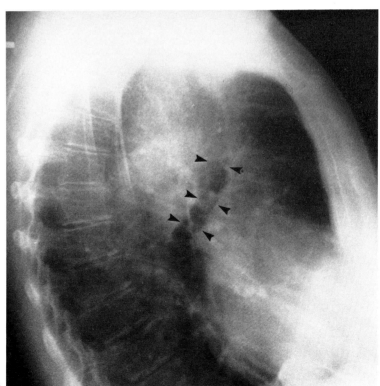

B

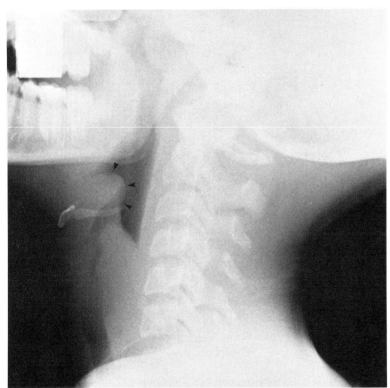

Figure 7–18. Upper airway obstruction. **A.** Acute epiglottitis—markedly swollen epiglottis (*arrowheads*).

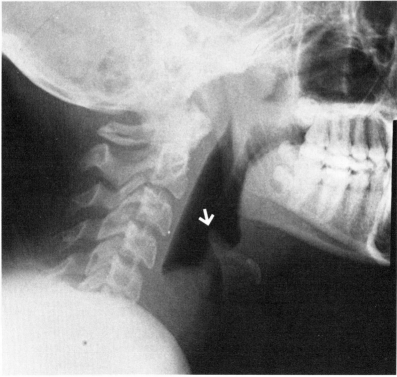

Figure 7–18B. Note almost normal epiglottis after 48 hours (*arrow*).

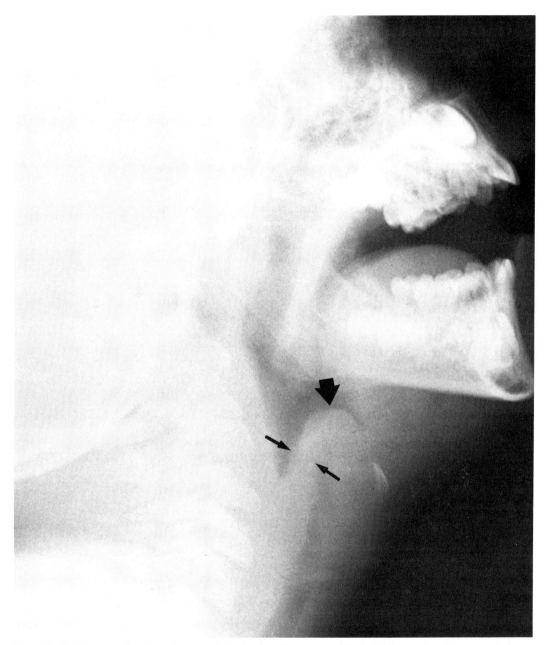

Figure 7–19. Obstructed trachea. Severe epiglottitis with edematous epiglottis (*wide arrow*) and aryepiglottis folds (*thin arrows*).

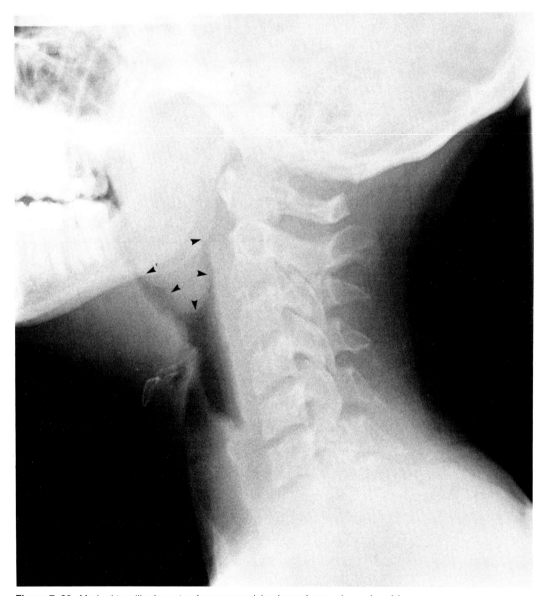

Figure 7–20. Marked tonsillar hypertrophy compromising hypopharynx (*arrowheads*).

Chapter 8

Trauma and Surgery

Lyle D. Victor, MD, *and Malcolm L. Weckstein*, MD

POSTTRAUMA CHEST ROENTGENOGRAPHY

The acutely injured patient often has major chest involvement, ranging from acute trauma of the chest wall to adult respiratory distress syndrome (ARDS). Fractures and blunt chest trauma are the injuries most frequently encountered in the critical care units.

Rib Fractures

Figure 8–1A shows a patient with fractured ribs associated with a pulmonary contusion. A contusion of the lung, like contusions of other body tissues, represents an area of acute traumatic inflammation containing a dense collection of clotted blood, leukocytes, and fibrin. Healing is eventually effected by clearance of the detritus and, in some cases, scarring. Figure 8–1B shows a close-up of the left mid-lung infiltrates in the same patient. The infiltrates (*asterisks*) are actually the x-ray film manifestations of lung contusions or hematoma. The *large arrow* shows distortion of a rib margin consistent with a rib fracture that occurred secondary to blunt trauma from an automobile accident. A roentgenogram of the same patient two weeks later (Fig. 8–1C) shows the healing rib fractures (*thin black arrows*). The contusions have resolved, but a residual hemothorax is present (*blunt arrows*). The hemorrhagic fluid layering

out posteriorly, forming a meniscus, is seen in Figure 8–1D. Blood in the pleural space should usually be removed, inasmuch as it has a tendency to cause scarring, pleural adhesions, and fibrothorax.

Trauma and contusion of the lung can result in traumatic lung cysts as shown by the *white arrows* in Figure 8–2. The infiltrative changes seen laterally represent the pulmonary contusions. Underlying rib fractures became more apparent a few weeks later—after healing of the lung had occurred.

Blunt Trauma

Massive trauma to the thoracic cage may cause a flail chest, clinically manifested by paradoxical movement of the damaged rib cage during respiration. The patient shown in Figure 8–3 received blunt trauma to the left hemithorax during a motor vehicle accident. The *arrowheads* delineate the multiple rib fractures that are present both anteriorly and posteriorly and allow the anterolateral chest cage to move freely inward on inspiration and outward on expiration (precisely the opposite occurs normally). Severe impairment of gas exchange causing hypoxemia and hypercarbia may also be present. The *large black arrow* points to a fractured clavicle; the thin arrows, to a chest tube placed for an associated pneumothorax; the *white arrows*, to subcutaneous emphysema.

Blunt trauma can also result in mediastinal hematoma (Fig. 8–4). Although these conditions frequently resolve spontaneously, one must always be concerned about associated trauma to the vital structures such as the trachea, esophagus, and great vessels (see Chapter 5).

Sternum Fracture

A fractured sternum is seen commonly as a result of the frequent performance of cardiopulmonary resuscitation. The patient shown in Figure 8–5A had had external cardiac massage after a cardiac arrest. When he awoke two days later, he complained of severe anterior chest pain. The lateral roentgenogram shows the fracture at the sternal-manubrial joint (*white arrows*). Another sternal fracture is seen in Figure 8–5B in a patient with osteoporosis who hit her anterior chest on a steering wheel. Such fractures usually heal spontaneously unless instability is present.

CHEST WALL ABNORMALITIES: SCOLIOSIS

Scoliosis is a condition in which the spine is twisted and laterally deviated. Such a condition is shown in Figure 8–6. Patients with severe scoliosis may develop restrictive ventilatory failure as they age because they experience compression of the lungs from the natural loss of vertebral height. The patient shown in Figure 8–6 was a massively obese scoliotic, who had CO_2 retention, polycythemia, and congestive heart failure. The *white arrows* point to the thoracic spine deviated far to the right. Associated atelectasis of the left lung (*asterisks*) is also present.

TRAUMATIC FOREIGN BODY

The patient shown in Figure 8–7 had his sternum penetrated by a drill bit during an industrial accident. The *arrows* point to a faint oblique opacity in Figure 8–7A. The actual sternal penetration is seen best on the lateral view (Fig. 8–7B).

THE POSTOPERATIVE CHEST ROENTGENOGRAM

Because bronchogenic carcinoma is the most common malignant neoplasm in males, the clinician in the critical care unit frequently sees chest films of patients who have undergone surgical lobectomy and pneumonectomy. Occasionally, a patient experiences such complications as are described below.

Figure 8–8A shows a chest roentgenogram taken immediately after a lobectomy. This film shows several features of the postoperative chest: the ribs appear more closely spaced because of loss of lung volume, there is residual blood and fluid at the right base (*asterisk*), and chest tubes have been placed intraoperatively for drainage. Figure 8–8B shows a postoperative chest film made several months after surgery. An empty space is seen where a rib was removed in order to perform a resection (*white arrows*). The diaphragm is somewhat elevated because of fibrosis and scarring.

Pneumonectomy

Figure 8–9A shows a postpneumonectomy chest roentgenogram. Again, an empty space is seen anteriorly and posteriorly where a rib was resected (*small white arrows*). The *large white arrow* points to the margin of resection where the fifth posterior rib has been resected. During lobectomy or pneumonectomy, one or more ribs may be removed, the fifth rib being the one most often resected.

An important roentgenographic feature after a pneumonectomy is the absence of vascular markings (due to a lack of lung tissue) in the resected hemithorax. Air fills the space initially, but later the area is gradually filled with fluid (Fig. 8–9B through 8–9D). Eventually, the area will fibrose and will be partially filled with some of the left-sided mediastinal contents (see also Fig. 8–10C).

Bronchopleural Fistula

A bronchopleural fistula is a connection between a bronchus and the pleural space. Air, secretions, fluid, or pus may then fill the pneumonectomy cavity. Figure 8–10 shows a typical sequence of events in the development of a bronchopleural fistula. Figure 8–10A shows a centrally located bronchogenic carcinoma (*white arrows*). Figure 8–10B, taken just after a total pneumonectomy, shows a typical empty hemithorax. The *arrows* point to subcutaneous air, a residual after chest tube removal. Figure 8–10C, taken nine months later, shows the hemithorax, opacified by fibrosis and scarring. Note that the trachea and the heart have shifted to the right to help fill the space created by lung removal, and hyperexpansion of the left lung has occurred. Figure 8–10D, taken one month later, now shows the presence of air and fluid because of the breakdown of the bronchial stump from progressive carcinomatous infiltration in the area. Note that there has been a partial return of the heart and the mediastinum to a near-normal position. Ambient air has entered the hemithorax because of the direct connection between the bronchus and the pleural space. This tract is known as a bronchopleural fistula.

Thoracoplasty

Years ago, one of the treatments for tuberculosis was thoracoplasty, a surgical procedure whereby the upper lobe or other lobes involved with tuberculosis were collapsed by actually caving in the chest wall (Fig. 8–11). The lowering of oxygen tensions thus created an inimical environment for growth of the tubercle bacillus. Thoracoplasty is usually an incidental finding on a chest roentgenogram, although some patients may have problems with a worsening of preexisting lung disease because of the added restrictive impairment thoracoplasty causes.

REFERENCES

Post-operative chest radiography. *AJR* 1980; 134:533.

Chest Disease Syllabus, American College of Radiology, pp 263–268.

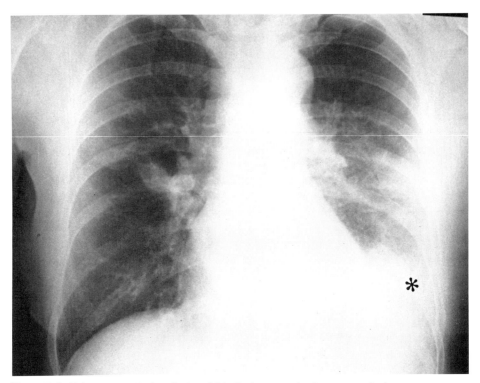

Figure 8–1. Pulmonary contusion. **A.** *Asterisk* indicates area of pulmonary contusion.

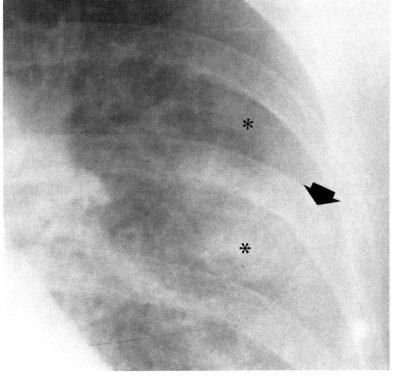

Figure 8–1B. In this closeup of film, *arrow* indicates rib fracture, and *asterisks* indicate area of pulmonary contusion.

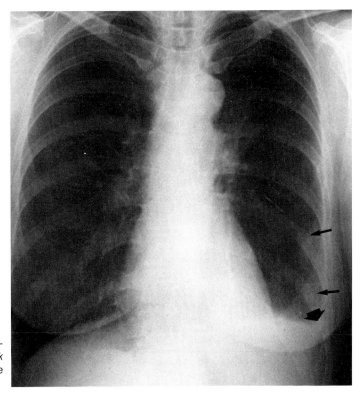

Figure 8–1C. *Thin black arrows* indicate healing rib fracture; *thicker black arrow* indicates fluid (blood) in the pleural space.

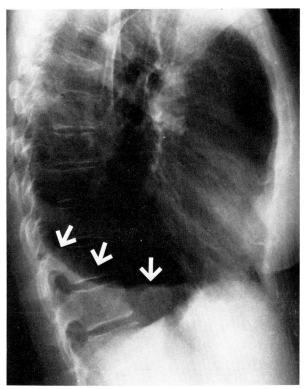

Figure 8–1D. Lateral view shows blood in the pleural space, forming a meniscus (*white arrows*).

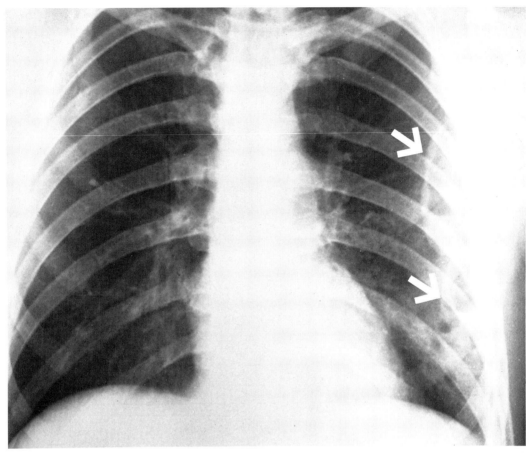

Figure 8–2. Posttraumatic lung cysts. *White arrows* delineate traumatic lung cysts; infiltrates in left lung represent contusions.

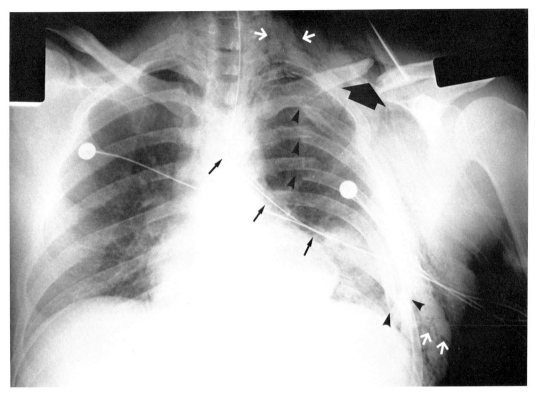

Figure 8–3. Flail chest. *Large black arrow* indicates fractured clavicle; *small black arrows* delineate a chest tube; *black arrowheads* show rib fractures; and *small white arrows* indicate areas of subcutaneous emphysema.

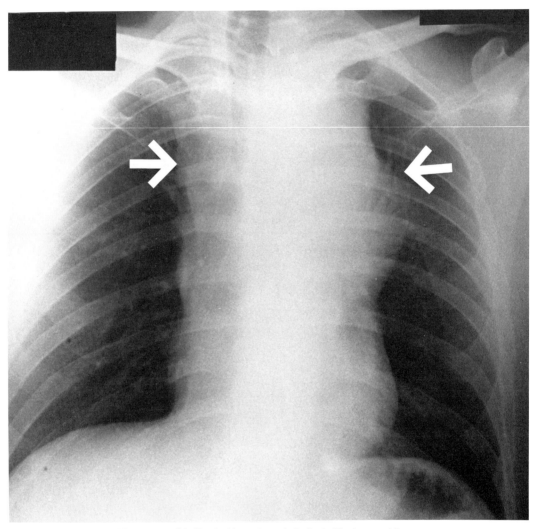

Figure 8–4. Mediastinal hematoma. Mediastinal hematoma is indicated by *large white arrows*.

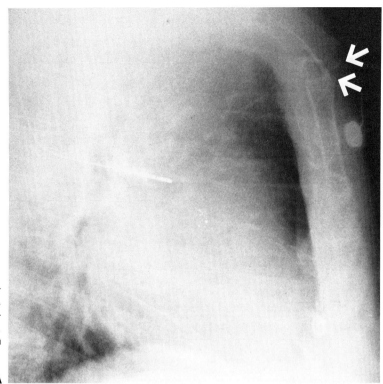

Figure 8–5. Fractured sternum: postresuscitation. **A.** Fractured sternum is delineated by *small white arrows*. **B.** Note fractured sternum (*white arrow*).

A

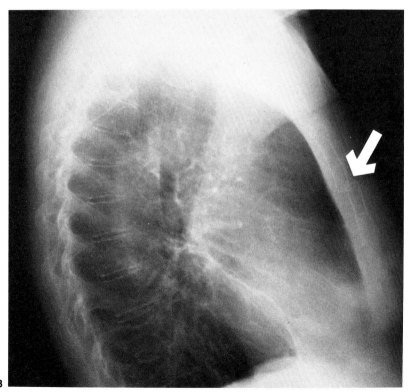

B

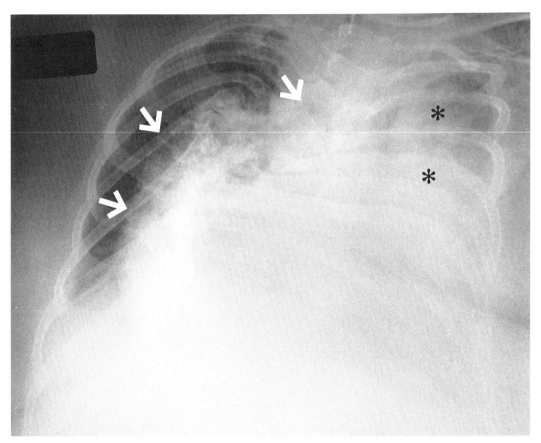

Figure 8–6. Scoliosis. Scoliosis of spine with convexity to right is delineated by small *white arrows*; *asterisks* indicate atelectasis of left lung.

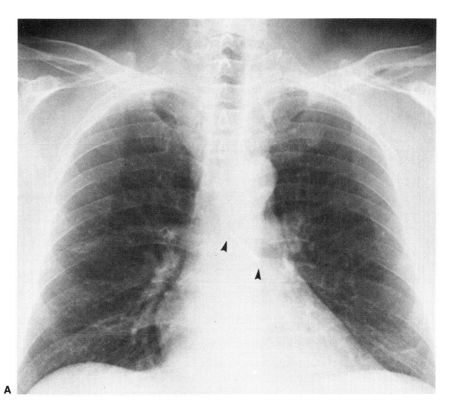

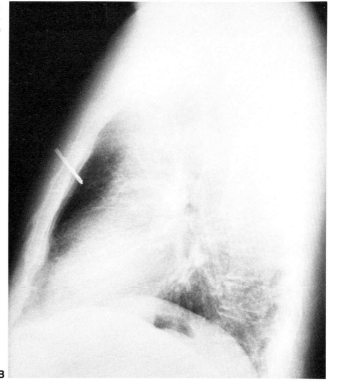

Figure 8–7. Foreign body in chest. **A.** In this PA view of chest, *black arrowheads* show drill bit in sternum. **B.** Lateral view of drill bit in sternum.

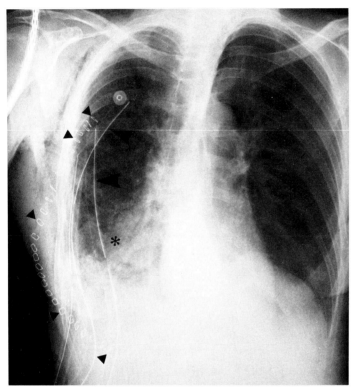

Figure 8–8. Postpneumonectomy. **A.** Immediate postoperative film shows surgical clips (*small arrowheads*), chest tubes (*large arrowheads*), and pleural effusion (*asterisk*).

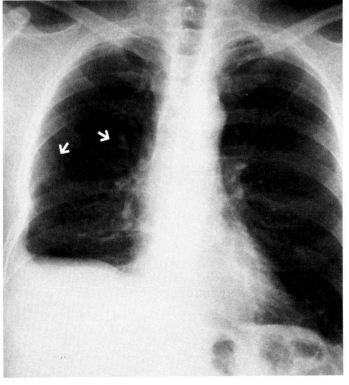

Figure 8–8B. Late postoperative film shows missing rib on right (*arrows*). Elevated right hemidiaphragm reflects loss of volume secondary to reduction in lung parenchyma.

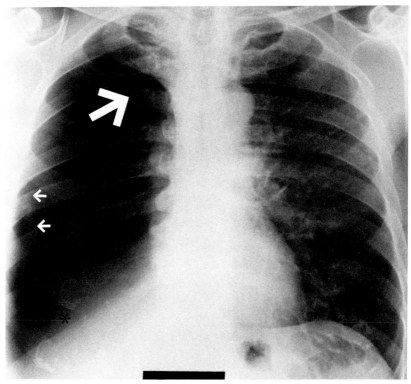

Figure 8–9. Postpneumonectomy. **A.** *Large arrow* shows residual posterior end of right fifth rib, *small arrows* show space left by resected rib, and *asterisk* indicates flattening of diaphragm.

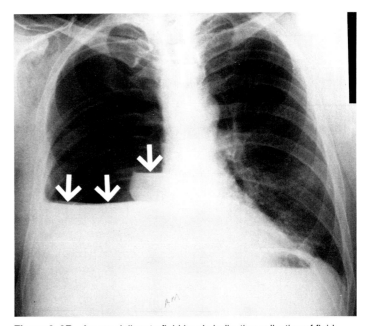

Figure 8–9B. *Arrows* delineate fluid levels indicating collection of fluid.

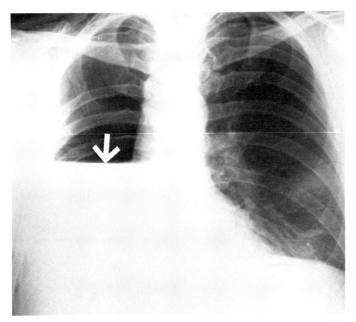

Figure 8–9C. *Arrow* indicates increase in fluid since prior film (Fig. 8–9B).

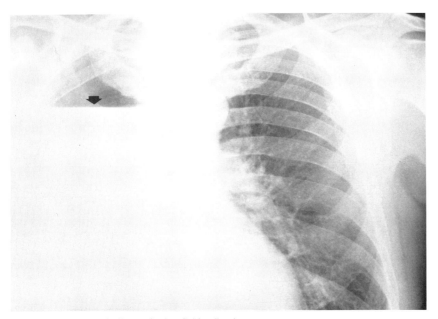

Figure 8–9D. *Arrow* indicates further fluid collection.

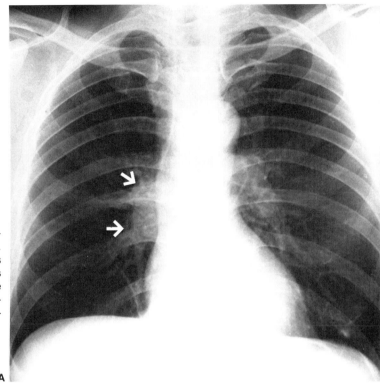

Figure 8–10. Pneumonectomy for lung cancer. **A.** *Arrows* delineate hilar mass before surgery. **B.** Film shows immediate postoperative period. Note empty right hemithorax; *arrows* show subcutaneous emphysema.

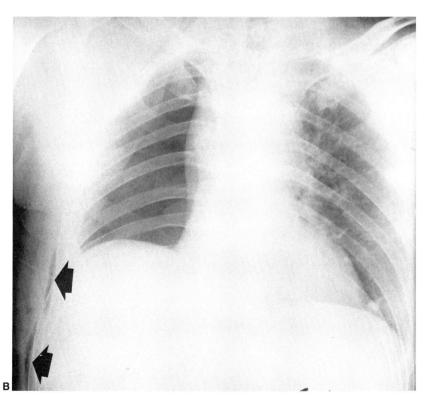

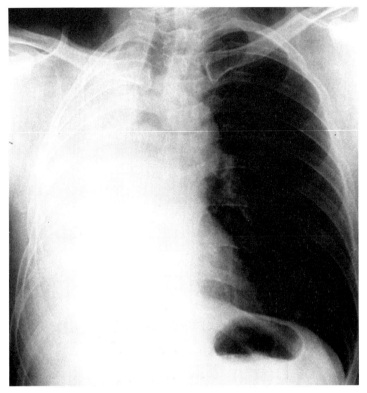

Figure 8–10C. Note total opacification of right hemithorax from fibrosis.

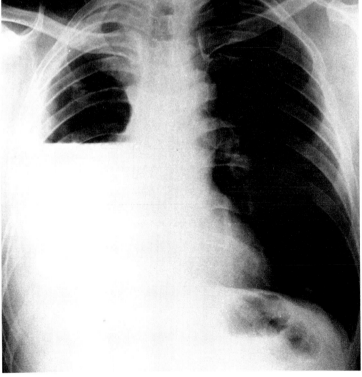

Figure 8–10D. Bronchopleural fistula has developed; note air-fluid level.

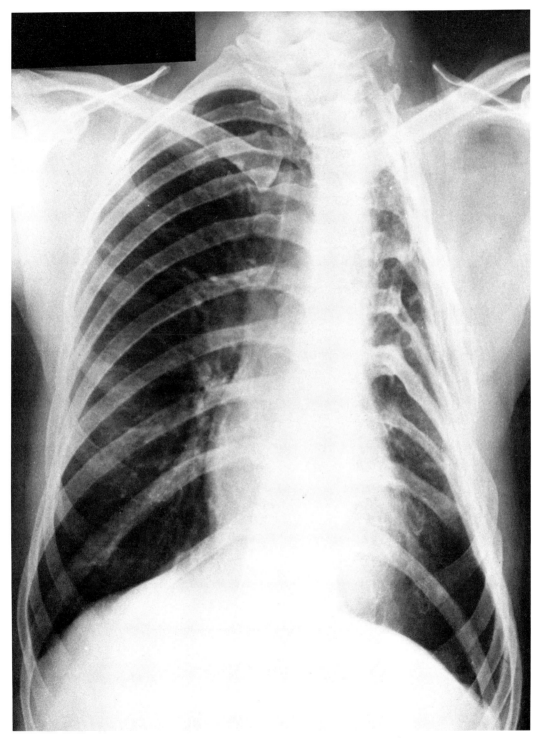

Figure 8–11. Thoracoplasty. Note left sided rib collapse (secondary to thoracoplasty).

Chapter 9

Critical Care Abdominal Roentgenography

Lyle D. Victor, MD, *Elias M. Mendoza,* MD, *and David Yates,* MD

Abdominal pathology may be identified on the chest roentgenogram because the abdominal contents are often visible on the standard portable antero-posterior (AP) chest film. In fact, the first indication of an acute abdomen may be seen during routine critical care chest roentgenography. Some of the common acute abdominal abnormalities are described below.

THE STANDARD ABDOMINAL FILM

The standard abdominal film ("flat plate") is shown in Figure 9–1. The superior aspect of the abdomen is delineated by the diaphragm, whereas the inferior aspect is bordered by the pelvic bones. The hazy area just beneath the dome of the right hemidiaphragm is the liver. The stomach is recognized as a collection of gas within the left upper quadrant beneath the left hemidiaphragm. Further abdominal gas is found in the large bowel. Little or no gas is normally seen within the small bowel. Different anatomic locations and bowel gas patterns differentiate them physically and geographically. The large bowel has haustral markings, which are lateral indentations evolving from the bowel's edge and extending partially across the lumen of the bowel (Fig. 9–2A; *large arrows*). The small bowel has valvulae conniventes (*small arrows*); they are differentiated from the haustral markings in that they extend entirely around the bowel wall and occur in greater frequency. Another differentiat-

ing point is the relative paucity of air normally found in the small bowel except in disease states. The large bowel, on the other hand, often contains air mixed with feces, which appears as a speckled pattern. The renal margins as well as the psoas margins are frequently, at least partially, seen on the plain film of the abdomen.

THE PATHOLOGIC ABDOMINAL FILM

Small-Bowel Obstruction

Small-bowel obstruction is a common cause of acute abdominal pain and distention among patients in the critical care unit. Distended loops of bowel lined up in horizontal rows are the hallmark of obstruction.

One cause of small-bowel obstruction is the intestinal passage of a gallstone. Known as gallstone ileus, this condition is seen most often in middle-aged women who pass the stone through a cholecystenteric fistula that communicates with the duodenum and, more rarely, the colon. The stone can usually pass relatively easily until it reaches the ileum, where obstruction often occurs. Figure 9–2B shows the typical roentgenographic pattern of small-bowel obstruction in this disorder. The *black arrow* points to air in the biliary tree caused by a fistula with the duodenum. Distended loops of small bowel are lined up in rows with typical elongated contours (*white arrows*).

Large-Bowel Obstruction

Large-bowel obstruction generally shows a wide distention of the bowel lumen; the prominent haustral markings do not circumscribe the lumen. Abrupt termination of gas at the point of obstruction is a frequent finding, although there may be air in the rectal ampulla. Figure 9–3A demonstrates sigmoid colon obstruction (*open arrow*). A barium enema was employed (Fig. 9–3B) to demonstrate an incarcerated femoral hernia (*arrow*).

Gastric Dilatation

Normally, a small amount of air may be seen in the gastric fundus just beneath the left hemidiaphragm. Larger amounts of air (Fig. 9–4A), can be seen in several critical care situations, including air swallowing in the case of the hyperventilating patient in respiratory failure or esophageal intubation. A nasogastric tube can usually decompress the dilated viscus (Fig. 9–4B). Massive gastric dilatation can be life-threatening, because diaphragmatic movement can be compromised. Figure 9–5A is an abdominal roentgenogram of a 12-year-old retarded girl that was made after a presumed toxic substance ingestion. The *white arrows* show massive gastric distention. Partial decompression was effected by inserting a nasogastric tube (Fig. 9–5B). Unfortunately, perforation of the gastric antrum occurred and resulted in free intraperitoneal air underneath the right hemidiaphragm (*asterisks*).

Perforated Viscus

Perforation of the stomach or the bowel allows free air to enter the intraperitoneal or retroperitoneal spaces. There are several distinctive manifestations of free extraintestinal air. One common manifestation is free air underneath the diaphragm, a frequent location of free intraperitoneal air in the upright position because the air collects in a nondependent location due to gravity (Fig. 9–6A); the liver edge is marked by the *wide arrow* and the dome of the diaphragm by the *thin arrow*. In the same patient (Fig. 9–6B), *small arrows* point to the inside and outside of the bowel wall, which can be seen because of intraluminal and free intraperitoneal air. The *open arrow* points to air surrounding the falciform ligament. A normal intraluminal gas pattern is shown by the open circles.

Retroperitoneal air may outline the kidneys (Fig. 9–7). The patient had a perforated sigmoid colon after a rectal biopsy, resulting in air dissecting into the retroperitoneal space.

In situations causing bowel necrosis, gas may locate in the portal venous system (Figs. 9–8A and 9–8B). Necrosis of the bowel wall can lead to passage of intestinal gas into the bowel wall, leading to a condition known as pneumatosis intestinalis (Fig. 9–8B; *curved arrows*). Air may then enter the intestinal vasculature, eventually enter the portal venous system, and go on to the liver.

Subphrenic Abscess

Surgery and perforation of a viscus are situations that may lead to peritoneal infection. These infections have a predilection for the subdiaphragmatic space, the majority occurring on the right side. The infections are collectively known as subphrenic abscesses. The roentgenogram of a patient who suffered a perforated gastric fundus is seen in Figure 9–9. Several distinctive features of subphrenic abscess can be noted. Air-fluid level occurs beneath the right hemidiaphragm, likely secondary to growth of gas-forming bacteria (*open arrow*). Pleural effusion, which is usually called a sympathetic effusion, is also present (*white arrow*). It represents an exudate of fluid secondary to localized inflammation beneath the diaphragm. Finally, diffuse air-fluid levels are seen because of the associated ileus in this problem. A similar process is seen on the left side: fluid obliterates the left diaphragm and distance is increased between the lung and the gastric air bubble because of the inflammatory process and the pleural fluid (*arrowheads*).

Toxic Megacolon

Toxic megacolon is a complication of ulcerative colitis in which there is an acute massive distention of the colon. The etiology is unknown. Mortality can be as high as 30 percent. The transverse colon demonstrates the greatest distention in the supine patient, but the entire colon is usually involved. The bowel wall becomes extremely thin and shows pseudopolyps (Fig. 9–10; *black arrows*) and ulcerations (*curved arrows*). There is a threat of perforation; barium enema is contraindicated.

Ascites

An occasional cause of hypoventilatory respiratory failure is massive abdominal distention from ascites. The patient shown in Figure 9–11 had a perforated stomach and peritonitis with acute massive collection of abdominal fluid that appears roentgenographically as a diffuse increase in abdominal density, bulging flanks, and high diaphragm. The abdominal fluid created such restriction to diaphragmatic movement that an acute CO_2 retention and respiratory acidosis ensued, requiring mechanical ventilatory support.

Diaphragmatic Defects

Hiatal Hernia

Weakness in the diaphragmatic structures can allow herniation of the abdominal contents into the thoracic cavity. Herniation of the air-filled stomach—known as a hiatal hernia—can mimic an abscess (Fig. 9–12), but differentiation is relatively easy. In this case, there is the typical retrocardiac location of the hiatal hernia (Fig. 9–12B). Second, no thick radiodense inflam-

matory tissue surrounds the "cavity" like that frequently seen in abscess and infection. Third, reactive changes are not seen in the lung bases as one might expect in an abscess. Figures 9–12C and 9–12D demonstrate that the barium-filled hiatal hernia accounts for the mass shown on the chest films.

Traumatic Eventration

Acute abdominal trauma can physically damage the diaphragmatic musculature and allow abdominal contents to appear in a thoracic herniation. Figure 9–13 is a chest roentgenogram of a patient who received a heavy blow to the abdomen that caused a tear in the diaphragm and which allowed a portion of the liver underneath the weakened diaphragm to herniate superiorly into the thoracic cavity (*arrowhead*).

Sengstaken-Blakemore Tubes

The Sengstaken-Blakemore tube is placed in cases of severe bleeding from esophageal varices. Consisting of a flexible plastic tube with an inflatable balloon on the distal tip, it is placed in the stomach. Air is then blown into the balloon, and the tube is pulled back, exerting pressure against the gastroesophageal junction, in hopes of tamponading the esophageal bleeding (Fig. 9–14). An esophageal balloon is situated proximal to the gastric balloon. It is inflated if the gastric balloon does not halt the variceal bleeding.

REFERENCES

Marshak, R.: *Radiology of the Colon.* Philadelphia, WB Saunders, 1980.

Margulis, A, Burhenne, HJ: *Acute Ulcerative Colitis.* Alimentary Tract Radiology, ed. 3. St. Louis, C.V. Mosby Co., 1983, Vol 1, pp 407–410.

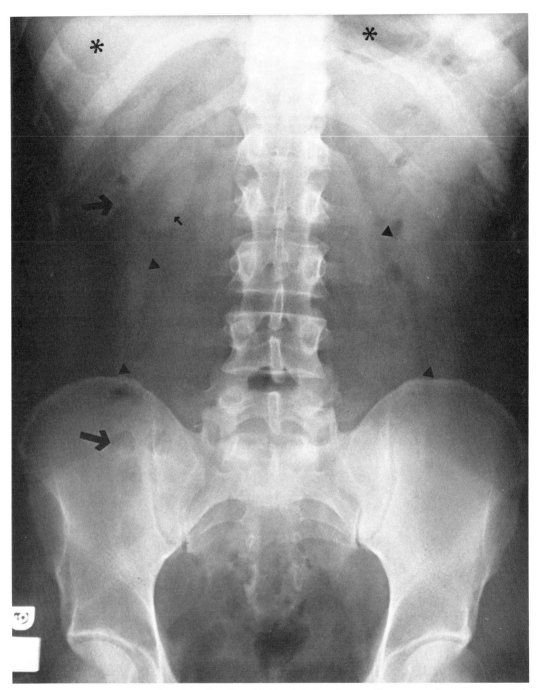

Figure 9–1. Normal abdominal flat plate. Note liver (*right asterisk*), colon gas (*large arrows*), stomach gas (*left asterisk*), psoas margins (*arrowheads*), and renal margins (*small arrow*).

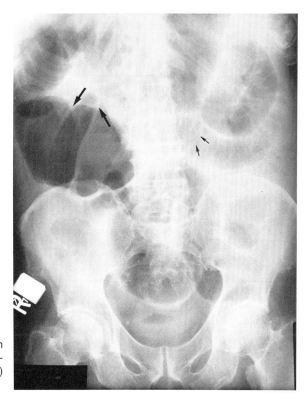

Figure 9–2. Bowel gas patterns. **A.** Patient with adynamic ileus demonstrates valvulae conniventes in dilated small-bowel loops (*small arrows*) and haustral markings in colon (*large arrows*).

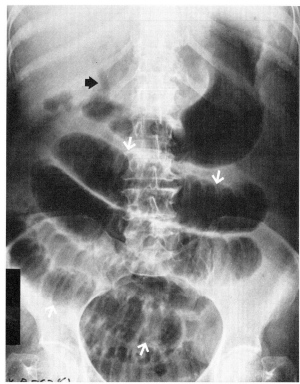

Figure 9–2B. Another patient with small-bowel obstruction due to gallstone ileus. Note air in biliary tree (*black arrow*) and dilated loops of small bowel (*white arrows*).

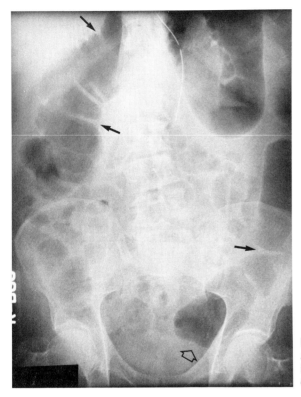

Figure 9–3. Patient with distal colon obstruction. **A.** Note dilated proximal colon with haustral markings (*arrows*) and abrupt termination at point of obstruction (*open arrow*).

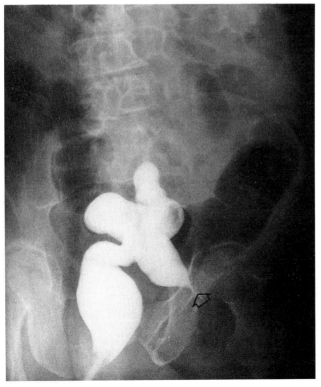

Figure 9–3B. Barium enema on same patient shows point of obstruction, an incarcerated hernia (*arrow*).

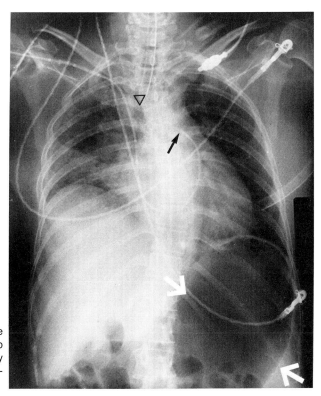

Figure 9–4. Gastric dilatation. **A.** Note acutely dilatated viscus (*white arrows*); also note Swan-Ganz catheter in left pulmonary artery outflow tract (*black arrow*) and endotracheal tube (*arrowhead*).

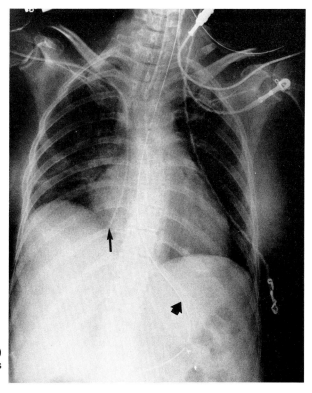

Figure 9–4B. Nasogastric tube (*wide arrow*) has decompressed stomach; *thin arrow* shows tip of central venous catheter in right atrium.

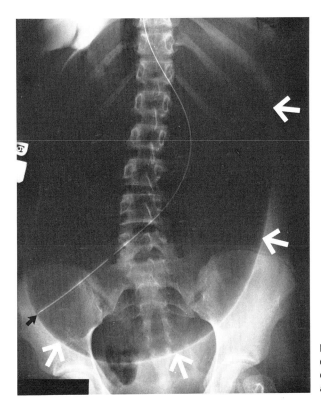

Figure 9–5. Gastric dilatation. **A.** Note massive distention (*white arrows*) due to gastric outlet obstruction; nasogastric tube is present (*black arrow*).

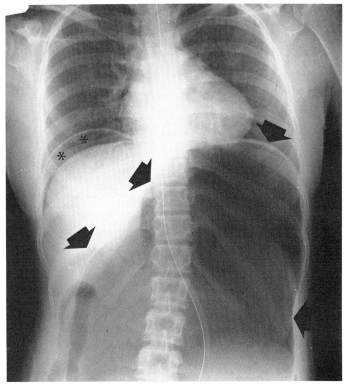

Figure 9–5B. Same patient with massive gastric distention (*black arrows*); note evidence of perforation with free air under right hemidiaphragm (*asterisks*).

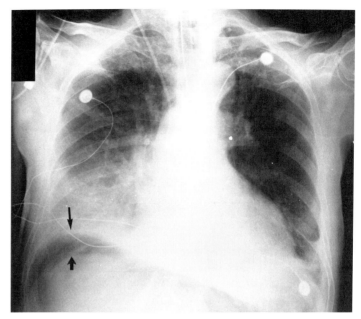

Figure 9–6. Perforated viscus. **A.** Note resultant air under right hemidiaphragm; *thin arrow* points to diaphragm and *wide arrow* to liver margin.

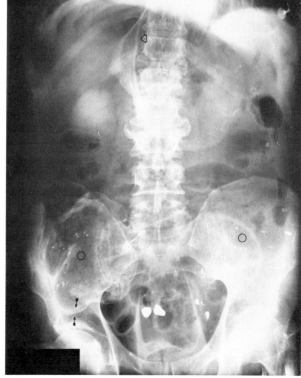

Figure 9–6B. Note air inside and outside of bowel wall (*thin arrows*); intraluminal bowel gas (*circles*), and falciform ligament (*open arrow*).

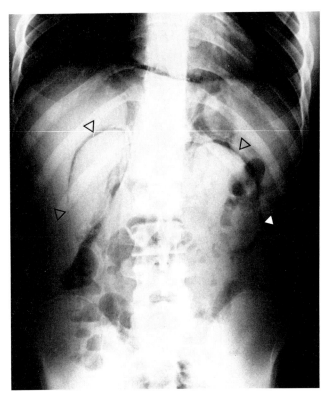

Figure 9–7. Retroperitoneal air. Air can be seen outlining kidneys (*white arrowheads*).

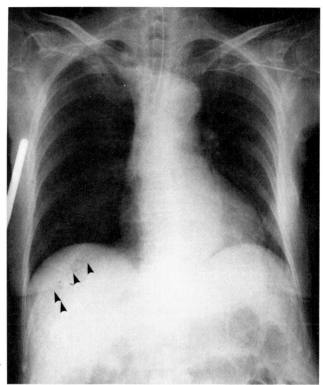

Figure 9–8. Bowel necrosis gas. **A.** Note air in portal venous system (*arrowheads*).

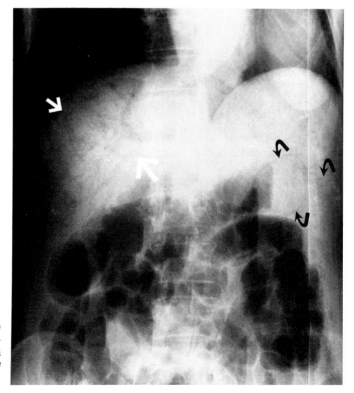

Figure 9–8B. Streaks of air can be seen within portal vein (*arrows*). Pneumatosis intestinalis or air in bowel wall is associated with bowel necrosis (*curved arrows*).

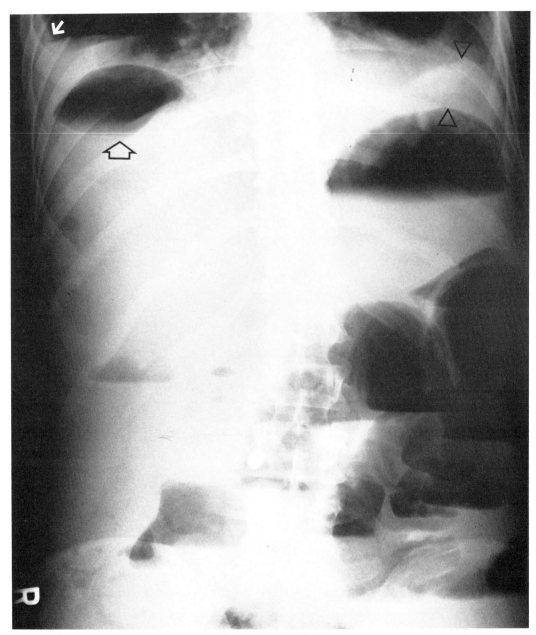

Figure 9–9. Patient with subphrenic abscess. Note air fluid level in right upper quadrant (*open arrow*), right pleural effusion (*arrow*), and left pleural effusion (*arrowheads*).

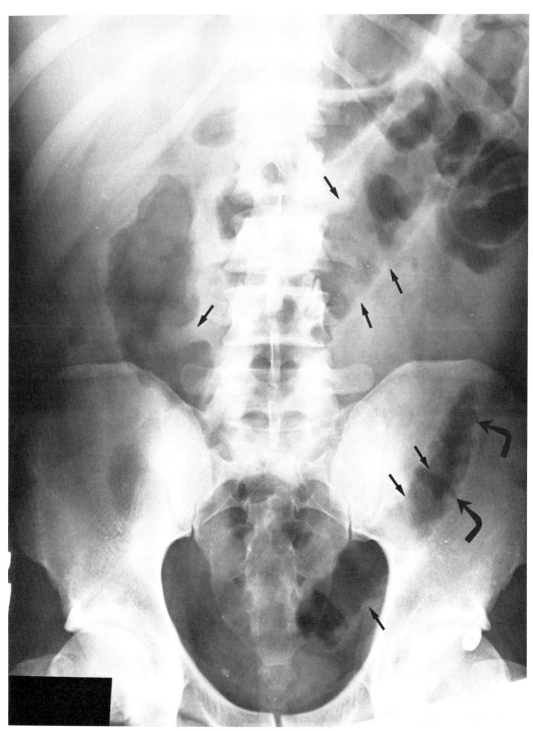

Figure 9–10. Toxic megacolon. *Straight arrows* point to pseudopolyps of colon; *curved arrows* demonstrate deep ulcerations.

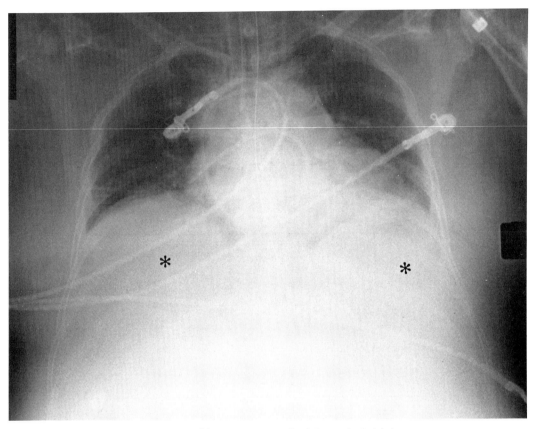

Figure 9–11. Massive ascites gives overall hazy appearance to abdomen (*asterisks*).

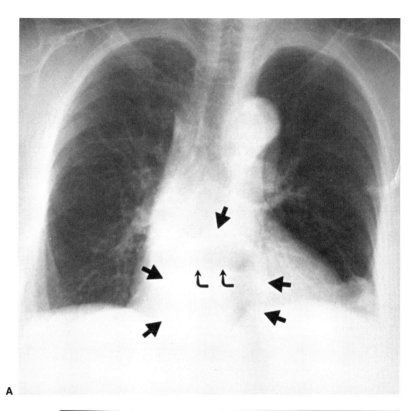

A

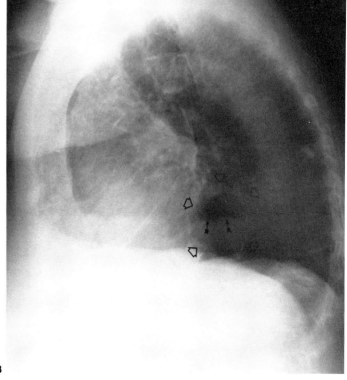

B

Figure 9–12. Hiatal hernia. **A.** "Mass" (*large arrows*) with an air-fluid level (*curved arrows*) is superimposed over the heart. **B.** Lateral film demonstrates typical retrocardiac location of hiatal hernia (*open arrows*); air-fluid level is shown by *arrows*.

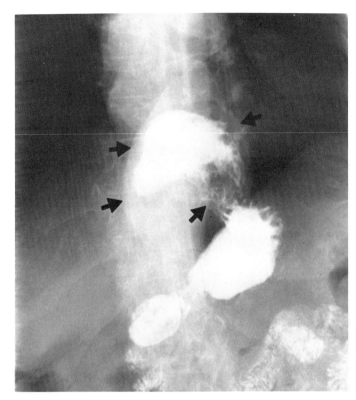

Figure 9–12C. Barium swallow. Hiatal hernia containing gastric fundus (*arrows*) corresponds to mass shown in Figure 9–12A. There is no air-fluid level because patient is supine.

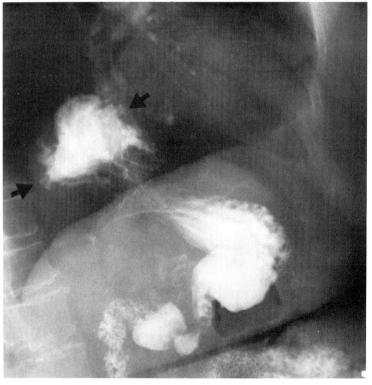

Figure 9–12D. Lateral film demonstrates hiatal hernia in retrocardiac location.

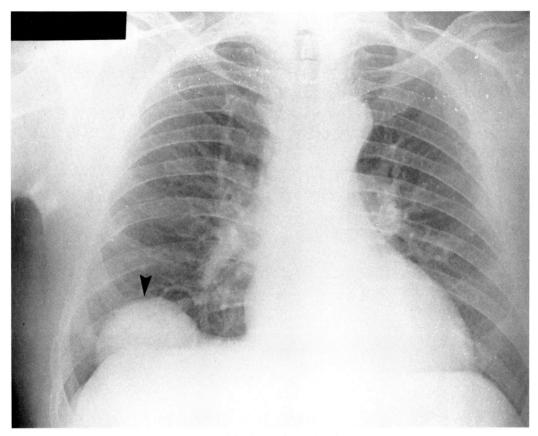

Figure 9–13. Localized traumatic eventration of diaphragm (*arrowhead*).

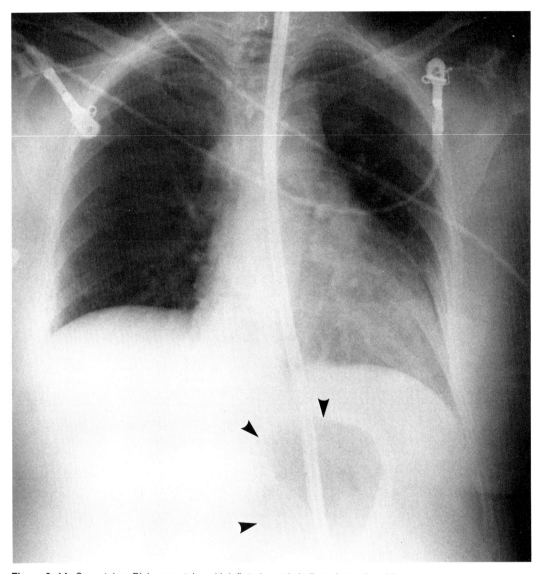

Figure 9–14. Sengstaken-Blakemore tube with inflated gastric balloon (*arrowheads*).

Chapter 10

Neonatal Chest Roentgenography

Allen J. Stone, MD

The majority of infants in the neonatal intensive care unit suffer from some form of respiratory distress that must be closely monitored with chest roentgenography. The chest film functions as a watchdog for a close assessment of the status of the lungs and the pleural space. Many of the respiratory complications occurring secondary to mechanical ventilation can be demonstrated early on chest roentgenography.

THE NORMAL NEONATAL CHEST FILM

The cardiothymic shadow comprises 60% to 65% of the transverse diameter of the neonatal chest. The thymus gland occupies the anterior mediastinum extending from the thoracic inlet to the cardiac margins (Fig. 10–1A; *blunt arrows*). Because of its anterior location, the thymus obscures the margins of the heart. The inferior portion of the thymus creates a notch with the heart margin (*thin black arrow*). The thymus gland becomes smaller on inspiration and during stressful situations. Figures 10–1A and 10–1B demonstrate a decrease in the size of the thymus over a period of two days due to the stress of hypoxia. The lateral view of the chest clearly demonstrates that the thymus occupies the retrosternal space (Fig. 10–1C; *arrow*). Because there is shrinkage of the thymus following stress, the retrosternal air space can be observed (Fig. 10–1D; *arrows*).

The thymus gland can also appear as a unilateral superior mediastinal triangular structure,

mimicking a mass or consolidation (Fig. 10–2A; *asterisk*). This condition is called the *sail sign*. Note the undulation of the lateral margin of the thymus, referred to as the thymic wave sign (*arrows*). This irregular contour is present because of the approximation of the thymus to the anterior ribs. The lateral view (Fig. 10–2B), demonstrates the sharp inferior margin of the thymus sail (*straight arrow*).

PATHOLOGIC NEONATAL CHEST FILMS

Hyaline Membrane Disease

Hyaline membrane disease (HMD) or respiratory distress syndrome of the newborn is a common etiology of respiratory distress in the neonatal intensive care unit. This disease is seen in premature infants who lack surfactant, a surface tension reducing lipoprotein. The resultant increase in alveolar surface tension leads to collapse of the alveoli and reduced pulmonary compliance. Diffuse atelectasis and decrease in lung volume are also features of this disease. The clinical and radiologic features are manifest within three or four hours of birth. These neonates are hypoxic and in severe respiratory distress. The roentgenogram reveals a diffuse granularity with decreased volume (Fig. 10–3A). Air bronchograms (*blunt arrows*) are demonstrated. They extend peripherally and are surrounded by the opacified lung parenchyma.

In the past, most of these infants died within a few days of birth. The survival rate reaches 80 percent in modern neonatal intensive care units with neonatologists and sophisticated equipment. The lungs in cases of HMD have a low compliance and require high ventilatory pressures to ventilate with an adequate tidal volume. These high pressures can cause air to rupture through the alveoli into the perivascular sheaths and interlobular septa causing pulmonary interstitial emphysema (PIE). Figure 10–3B demonstrates unilateral PIE on the right characterized by cysts or "bubbles" (*black arrows*) and air-filled streaks (see also Fig. 10–4; *blunted arrows*), which do not branch or taper. It is important to recognize this condition because the lungs become less compliant and present an imminent threat of pneumothorax. PIE may give a false radiographic impression of improvement because the interstitial air decreases the opacification of the lung. For example, the patient shown in Figure 10–3 developed a tension pneumothorax (Fig. 10–3C) a short time later. Note the depression of the right hemidiaphragm and the shift of the mediastinum to the contralateral side.

PIE can also be manifested by one or more subpleural cysts (Fig. 10–4; *large arrows*). Pneumomediastinum can also be a complication of PIE. The air in the perivascular sheaths can dissect medially into the mediastinum. Figure 10–5 demonstrates that the thymus gland (*white arrows*) has been carried into the left lateral hemithorax by mediastinal air (*white arrows*). This peripheral location of the thymus is called the *spinnaker sign* of mediastinal emphysema. Figure 10–6 displays the bat-wing or angel-wing sign of pneumomediastinum, characterized by bilateral elevation of the thymus (*arrows*).

Bronchopulmonary Dysplasia

HMD can eventually progress to bronchopulmonary dysplasia (BPD) in a high percentage of cases. Whether this condition is due to prolonged mechanical ventilation or to high oxygen concentration is controversial.

In the initial stage of BPD, the lungs become more opaque because of pulmonary edema. In the next few weeks cystlike changes occur. These cysts are caused by marked expansile changes in the alveoli. Figure 10–7A demonstrates an infant with classic HMD who, after several weeks of intubation, developed BPD (Fig. 10–7B), characterized by numerous cystic changes (*arrows*) and overexpansion of both lungs. Six months later (Fig. 10–7C), chronic changes of bronchopulmonary dysplasia, characterized by fibrotic strands radiating from the hila on the left (*arrows*) and bulla formation (*asterisks*), are demonstrated.

Patent Ductus Arteriosus

Hypoxia associated with HMD can cause a patent ductus arteriosus (PDA) resulting in a left to right shunt into the pulmonary arteries. This condition can lead to pulmonary edema accompanied by biventricular and left atrial enlargement. Because of the large shunt, a murmur may not be present. The radiologic changes may be subtle because of the underlying pulmonary disease. However, an increase in pulmonary density due to pulmonary edema as well as the cardiac enlargement should strongly suggest the diagnosis.

Figure 10–8A demonstrates consolidative changes in both lungs which are shown to have increased in density (Fig. 10–8B). An increase in cardiac size has also occurred. A thoracotomy was performed and a metallic clip was placed on the ductus (Fig. 10–8C; *arrow*). Medical treatment has also been employed in some cases to promote closure of the ductus with antiprostaglandins such as indomethacin.

Transient Tachypnea of the Newborn

Infants who have transient tachypnea of the newborn (TTN) are usually delivered by cesarean section and so do not have the advantage of the fact that the vaginal birth canal compresses the thorax, thereby expressing fluid from the lungs. The respiratory distress is caused by the fluids retained in the lungs. The infant attempts to remove the fluid from the lungs through lymphatics and vascularity by grunting respirations. Roentgenographically, vascular congestion and lymphatic distention are characterized by streaking densities in the lungs (Fig. 10–9A; *curved arrows*). Pleural effusion (*long arrows*) and fluid in the minor fissure (*blunted arrow*) are displayed in this temporary disorder. There is also evidence of hyperaeration. These infants have positive radiographic and clinical findings for up to 48 hours becoming asymptomatic with negative roentgenograms at 72 hours (Fig. 10–9B).

Meconium Aspiration

Because respiratory activity is mild in the unstressed fetus the aspiration of amniotic fluid or meconium (fetal stool) is prevented. Oxygen deficit can cause intrauterine fetal distress, however, inducing defecation of meconium and deep respiratory gasps. The result is aspiration of amniotic fluid and meconium. The presence, then, of meconium in the fetal aspirate is proof of meconium aspiration. These infants are usually depressed, in severe respiratory distress, and postmature.

Roentgenographically, air trapping is seen because the aspirated particles cause distal bronchial obstruction. Patchy infiltrates may be seen throughout both lungs. The duration of abnormal findings depends on the ratio of amniotic fluid to meconium aspirate. The higher the ratio, the more rapid the clearing of infiltrate. Figure 10–10A demonstrates patchy consolidations in both lungs (*asterisks*), consistent with meconium aspiration. Treatment with oxygen and pulmonary toilet effected clearing within one day (Fig. 10–10B). Figure 10–11A also demonstrates patchy consolidation in both lungs (*asterisks*), which was diagnosed as meconium aspiration. Three days later (Fig. 10–11B), the patient developed a right-sided pneumothorax (*straight arrows*)—a common complication with meconium aspiration. Two days later (Fig. 10–11C), infiltrates (*asterisks*) are still observed in both lungs, indicating a high probability of a significant amount of meconium in the aspirate.

Neonatal Pneumonia

Infants with neonatal pneumonia can become infected in utero, during delivery, and after birth. Any number of causes have been implicated—including premature rupture of membranes, prolonged labor, placental infection, vaginal infection, and maternal fecal contamination during delivery. Nonhemolytic *streptococcus, Staphylococcus aureus,* and *Escherichia coli* are the most common organisms causing pneumonitis of the newborn. These infants have severe respiratory distress but are usually afebrile. The roentgenographic patterns are quite varied with diffuse nodularity, perihilar streaky densities, a diffuse hazy pattern as seen in hyaline membrane disease, and patchy infiltrates. Rarely, a lobar consolidation is seen. Figure 10–12 demonstrates a diffuse hazy pattern with a consolidative pattern in the right lower lobe.

Pulmonary Hemorrhage

Pulmonary hemorrhage is seen as a secondary complication of HMD, meconium aspiration, and other causes of hypoxia—especially in the premature neonate. Classically, bleeding is seen from the nose and the mouth. When hemorrhage occurs in the lung, the roentgenographic appearance is diffuse opacification of both lungs with air bronchogram (see Fig. 10–13; *arrow*). This pattern is similar to hyaline membrane disease.

Persistent Fetal Circulation

Persistent fetal circulation (PFC) can occur in the full-term infant because of the persistence of fetal pulmonary hypertension. There may be right to left shunting through the patent ductus, causing these infants to have cyanosis and respiratory distress. Roentgenographically, the lungs are hyperlucent because of the decreased vascularity (see Fig. 10–14). A secondary form of persistent fetal circulation can occur in a number of cardiac and respiratory abnormalities.

Congenital Lobar Emphysema

Some infants with a congenital defect may develop bronchial occlusion accompanied by a ball-valve type obstruction, which leads to a condition known as lobar emphysema. Many patients with congenital lobar emphysema are asymptomatic, although symptoms of dyspnea may occur in the postnatal period. The upper and middle lobes are the most commonly involved with this disorder. The obstruction is usually caused by underdevelopment of bronchial cartilage leading to collapse of the bronchus, but other mechanical causes can lead to the same disorder. The overaerated lobe compresses the adjacent lung and causes a contralateral shift of the mediastinum. Figure 10–15 demonstrates congenital lobar emphysema of the left upper lobe with compression atelectasis of the left lower lobe (*black arrow*). The mediastinum is shifted to the right, and the left hemidiaphragm is depressed by the emphysematous lobe. When symptomatic, this condition is best treated by lobectomy. The enlarged lobe may be opacified initially and may appear to represent a mass until the lobe eventually undergoes aeration.

Congenital Diaphragmatic Hernia

The congenital diaphragmatic hernia, which occurs lateral to the dorsal spine through the foramen of Bochdalek, may be a surgical emergency, inasmuch as some neonates having this condition are born with respiratory distress. Usually, hypoplasia of the ipsilateral lung and occasionally of the contralateral lung is present because of a shift of the mediastinum. The hernia more commonly occurs on the left side, with the intestine passing into the chest leading to a scaphoid abdomen. Roentgenographically, there are numerous round lucent areas of varying size representing bowel (Fig. 10–16; *circles*), with shift of the mediastinum into the opposite hemithorax. In this case, there is opacification of the right lung that may be caused by hypoplasia. These hernias may appear as an opacification until the bowel loops are aerated by the infant swallowing air. Clinically, bowel sounds can be auscultated in the chest.

Cystic Adenomatoid Malformation

Cystic adenomatoid malformation represents a hamartomatous malformation of a portion or all of a lung. This malformation is comprised of cysts lined with cells showing adenomatoid configurations. These cysts do not communicate directly with the bronchial tree but do receive air through collateral pathways. Initially, these masses may be solid; but shortly after birth, the cysts fill with air. If the malformation is large, it can cause respiratory distress and may be difficult to differentiate from a congenital diaphragmatic hernia. The presence of gas-filled bowel in the abdomen, however, rules out the latter. Figure 10–17 demonstrates a prominent lucent structure in the left lung (*arrows*) that represents a cystic adenomatoid malformation.

Unilateral Lung Agenesis

Unilateral pulmonary or lung agenesis can cause respiratory distress, although many infants with this condition have few or no symptoms. The pulmonary arteries and veins are absent, and the trachea continues directly into the bronchus of the normal lung. This abnormality may be associated with other congenital defects such as the tetralogy of Fallot. Radiologically, there is total opacification of the lung accompanied by hyperinflation of the normal lung and a shift of the mediastinum to the abnormal side (Fig. 10–18).

Hydrops Fetalis

A number of conditions such as erythroblastosis fetalis, cardiac arrhythmia, intrauterine infection, and congenital heart disease can lead to hydrops fetalis. Figure 10–19 demonstrates an infant with this condition characterized by diffuse soft-tissue edema (*large open arrows*), ascites causing diffuse abdominal hazy appearance, and pleural effusion (*small open arrows*). The prominent pleural effusions, along with ascites elevating the diaphragm, compromise respiratory activity.

Pleural Effusion

Isolated massive pleural effusion in the neonate is usually due to chylothorax (Fig. 10–20; *asterisk*). Chylothorax is thought to be caused by tearing of the thoracic duct during delivery. Others have felt that stretching of the duct or overdistention can cause leakage of chyle into the pleural space. Infants with pleural effusion can suffer from respiratory distress, which necessitates repeated thoracentesis or chest tube drainage. If these measures fail to stop the reaccumulation of this cloudy fluid, then a thoracotomy to ligate the thoracic duct may be necessary.

Malpositioned Endotracheal Tubes

Figures 10–21A and 10–21B demonstrate an endotracheal tube that was placed in the esophagus. The low placement on the frontal view and the posterior placement seen on the lateral view indicate esophageal placement. The endotracheal tube should be located at approximately the level of the first or second thoracic vertebral body. As is the case in the adult, it is easy to malposition the tube in the right mainstem bronchus of the neonate because of the inferior straight continuity of this bronchus (Fig. 10–22A). The following day, the tube has been properly positioned; however, the patient has a tension pneumothorax (*white arrows*) and a pneumomediastinum (*large white arrow*) caused by barotrauma from the previously malpositioned endotracheal tube (Fig. 10–22B).

REFERENCES

Caffey, J: *Pediatric X-Ray Diagnosis*, ed. 6. Chicago, Yearbook Medical Publishers, 1972, pp 1436–1477.

Swischuk, LE: *Radiology of the Newborn and Young Infant*, ed. 2. Baltimore, Williams & Wilkins, 1980, pp 1–189.

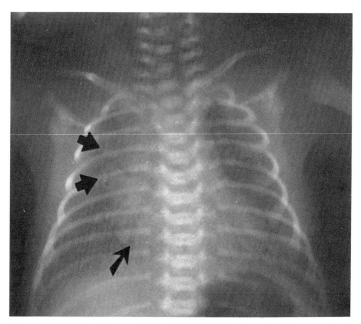

Figure 10–1. Normal neonatal chest. **A.** Note lateral margin of thymus gland (*blunt arrows*); cardiothymic notch demonstrates inferior margin of thymus (*thin arrow*).

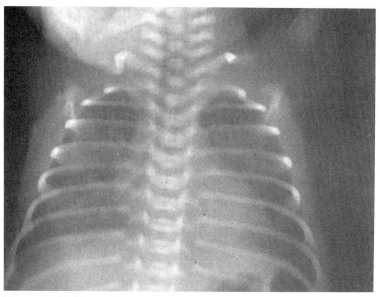

Figure 10–1B. Note marked decrease in size of thymus after hypoxia.

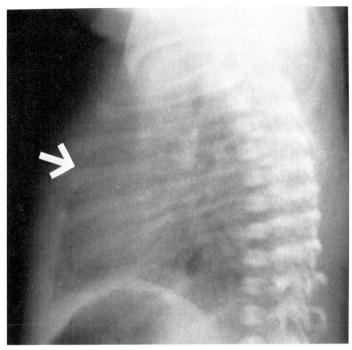

Figure 10–1C. Lateral view before hypoxic episode demonstrates thymus occupying retrosternal space (*white arrow*).

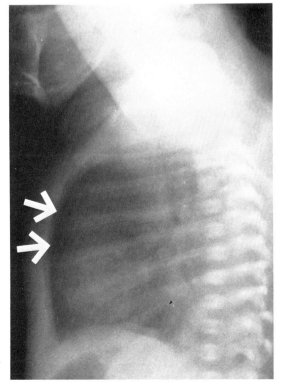

Figure 10–1D. Note decrease in thymic size with display of retrosternal air space (*white arrows*).

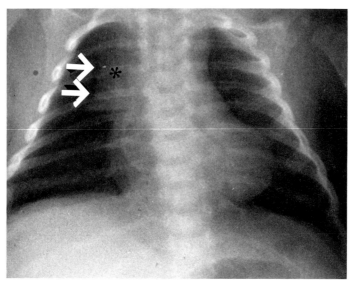

Figure 10–2. Thymic sail. **A.** Note triangular (sail) configuration of thymus gland (*asterisk*); lateral margin displaying undulation called thymic wave (*arrows*).

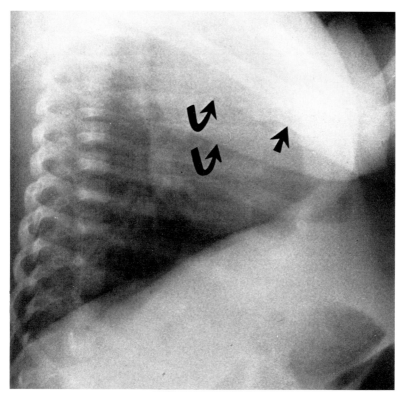

Figure 10-2B. Lateral film demonstrates inferior sharp margin of thymus gland (*straight arrow*). The soft tissues of both upper arms superimpose the chest (*curved arrows*).

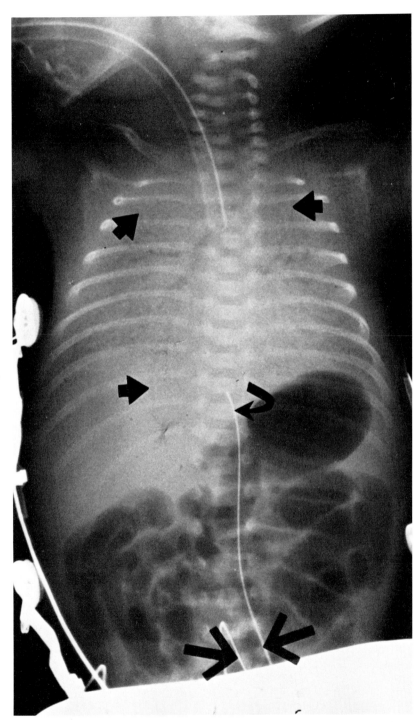

Figure 10–3. Hyaline membrane disease. **A.** Note diffuse consolidation with air bronchograms (*blunt arrows*) a few hours after birth. Umbilical arterial catheter loops as catheter descends to hypogastric artery and then turns up into the aorta (*large arrows*). The catheter ends at the level of the ninth dorsal vertebral body (*curved arrow*), well above the abdominal visceral arteries and below the aortic arch.

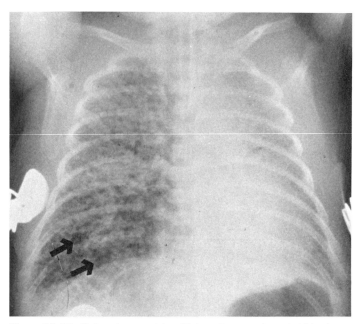

Figure 10–3B. Note pulmonary interstitial emphysema; large bubbles have now occurred following mechanical ventilation in HMD patient (*black arrows*).

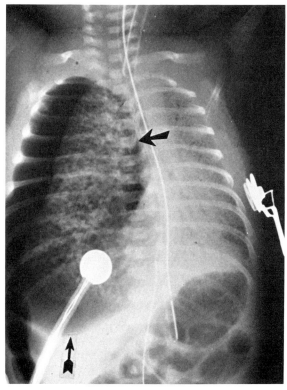

Figure 10–3C. Tension pneumothorax follows the interstitial emphysema with depression of right hemidiaphragm (*feathered arrow*) and contralateral shift of mediastinum (*straight arrow*).

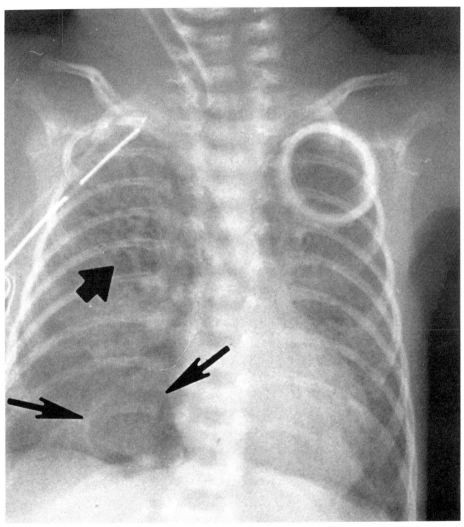

Figure 10–4. PIE with subpleural cyst. Large air streaks not branching (*blunt arrow*) and indicative of interstitial emphysema; round lucent area (*thin arrows*) points to subpleural interstitial cyst.

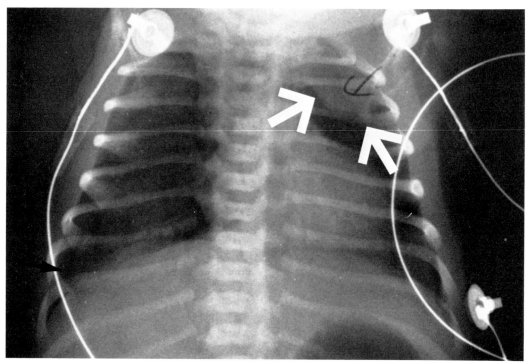

Figure 10–5. Pneumomediastinum. Condition is characterized by thymus gland deviated to left lateral chest wall causing spinnaker sign (*white arrows*); pneumothorax is on the right (*black arrow*).

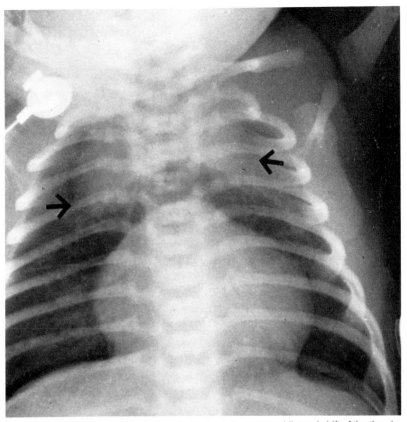

Figure 10–6. Pneumomediastinum. Mediastinal air causes a bilateral shift of the thymic lobes (*black arrows*) to form the bat-wing or angel-wing sign.

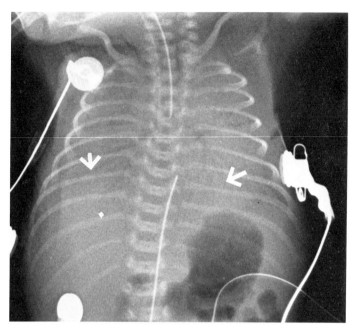

Figure 10–7. Bronchopulmonary dysplasia. **A.** Note HMD with diffuse consolidation and air bronchograms (*arrows*).

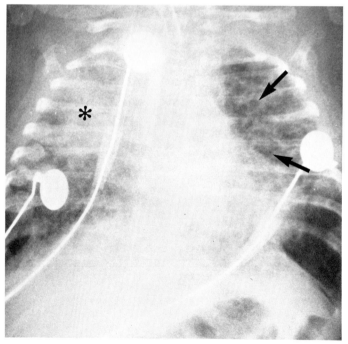

Figure 10–7B. Note bronchopulmonary dysplasia characterized by diffuse round cystic areas (*arrows*); area of consolidation is in right upper lobe (*asterisk*).

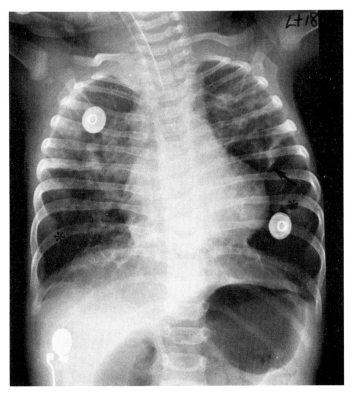

Figure 10–7C. Chronic changes of bronchopulmonary dysplasia with fibrotic strands extending from hila (*arrow*). Bulla formation is present in both lower lobes (*asterisk*).

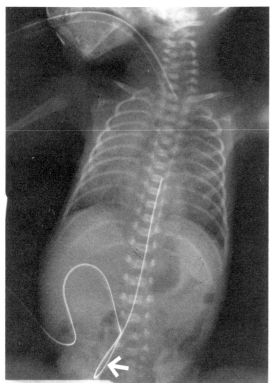

Figure 10–8. Patent ductus arteriosus. **A.** Note consolidative changes of HMD; also note loop of umbilical artery catheter (*arrow*).

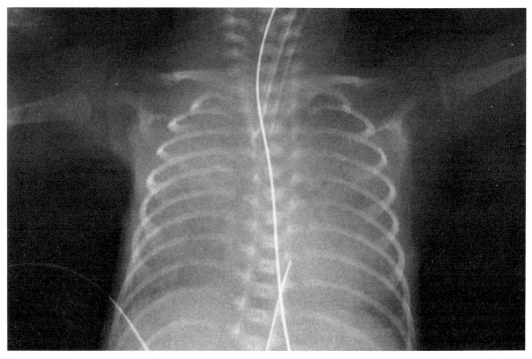

Figure 10–8B. Increasing opacification of both lungs is due to pulmonary edema. Increased heart size is also indicative of PDA.

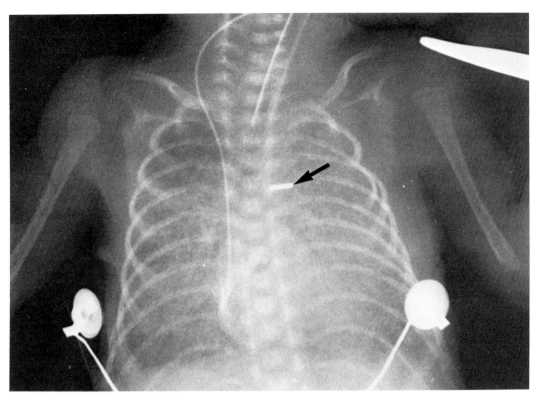

Figure 10–8C. Note postoperative clipping of ductus (*arrow*).

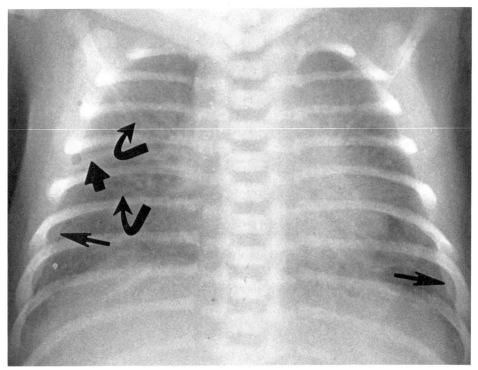

Figure 10–9. Transient tachypnea of the newborn. **A.** Note TTN with fluid in minor fissure (*blunt arrow*), basilar pleural fluid (*long arrows*), and streaking densities from hilum representing distended lymphatics and blood vessels (*curved arrows*).

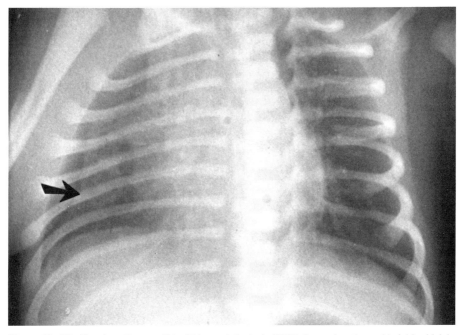

Figure 10–9B. Clearing of lungs within 48 hours is typical of TTN. *Arrow* denotes a skin fold, which is sometimes mistaken for pneumothorax.

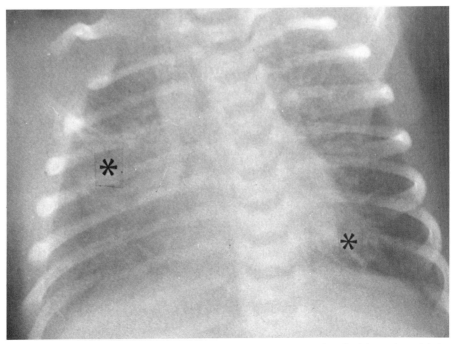

Figure 10–10. Meconium aspiration. **A.** Note patchy infiltrates throughout both lungs (*asterisks*).

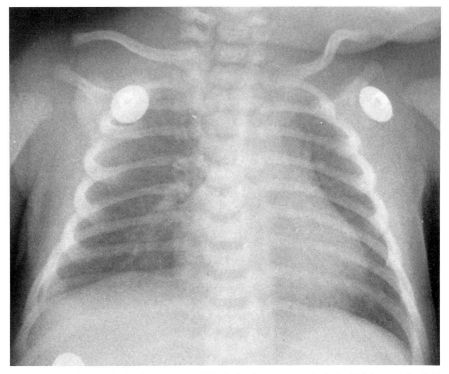

Figure 10–10B. Rapid clearing occurs within 1 day because aspirate had high amniotic fluid content relative to meconium.

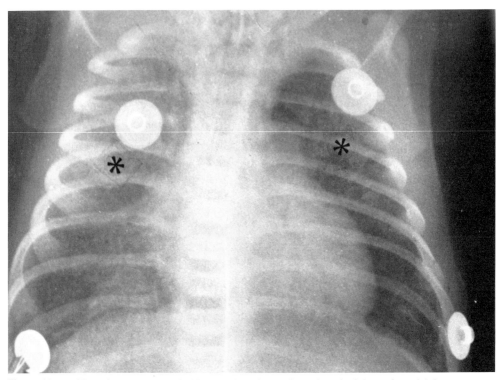

Figure 10–11. Meconium aspiration. **A.** Note patchy infiltrate throughout both lungs (*asterisks*).

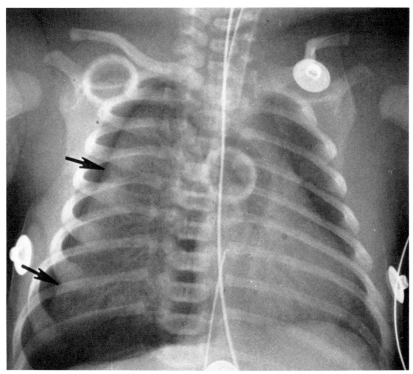

Figure 10–11B. Complicating tension pneumothorax has developed; *arrows* delineate visceral pleural line.

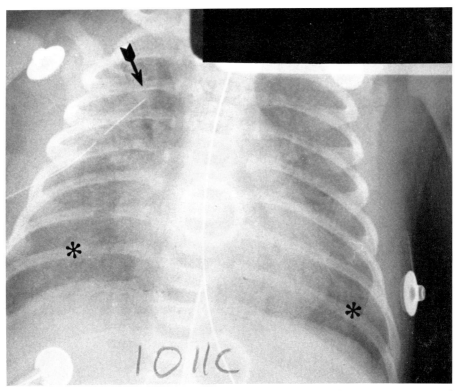

Figure 10–11C. Infiltrates (*asterisks*) persisting after several days favor greater amount of meconium in aspirate. *Arrow* indicates thoracotomy tube on right for treatment of pneumothorax.

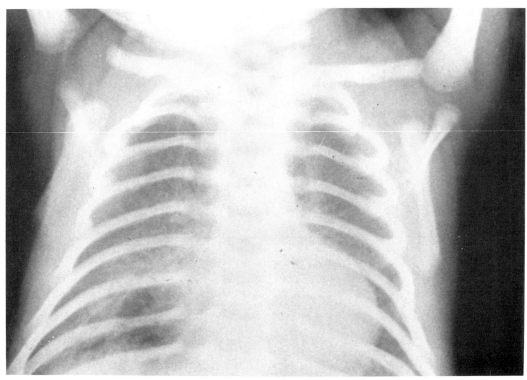

Figure 10–12. Neonatal pneumonia. Note diffuse hazy pattern of neonatal pneumonia with consolidative changes in right lower lobe.

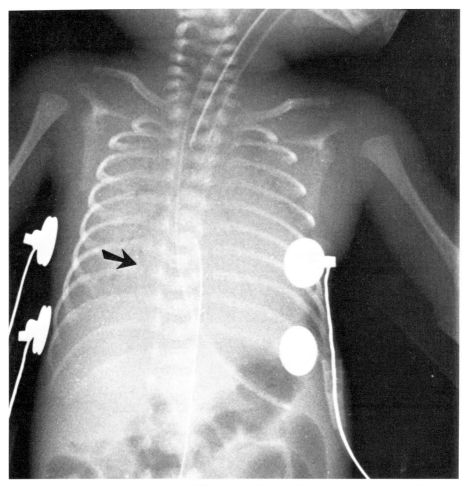

Figure 10–13. Pulmonary hemorrhage. Diffuse consolidation with air bronchogram (*arrow*) can be seen with diffuse pulmonary hemorrhage; note strong similarity to HMD. Neonatal pneumonia can also have this appearance.

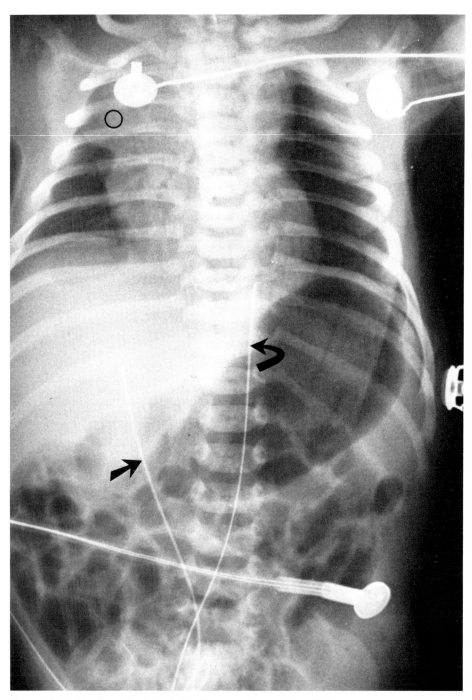

Figure 10–14. Persistent fetal circulation. Decreased vascularity of both lungs is due to pulmonary hypertension with right to left shunting. The solid density in right upper hemithorax is the thymus gland (*circle*). It is displayed far to the right because of the right-sided rotation of the patient. Note umbilical arterial catheter (*curved arrow*). Umbilical venous catheter (*straight arrow*) passes into portal venous system.

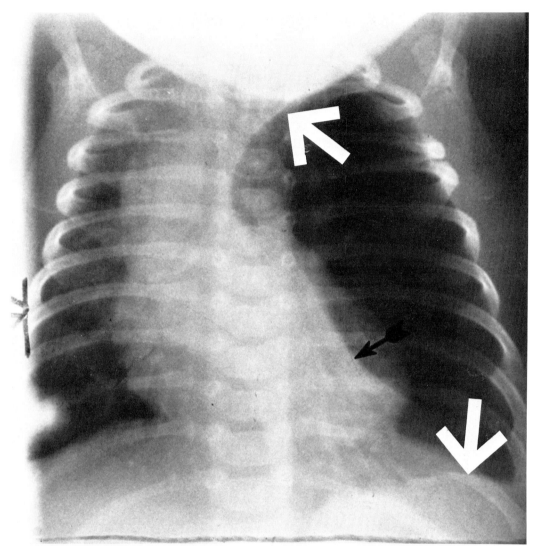

Figure 10–15. Congenital lobar emphysema. Expansile, hyperlucent, left upper lobe (*white arrows*) occupies entire left hemithorax. Left lower lobe is collapsed by emphysematous upper lobe (*black arrow*).

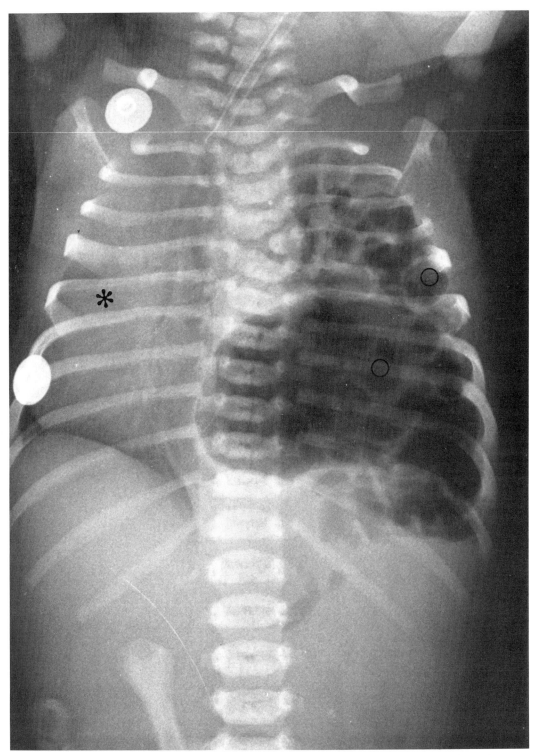

Figure 10–16. Congenital diaphragmatic hernia. The hernia is displayed on left side with multiple cystic areas representing gas-filled bowel (*circles*). There is a shift of the mediastinum to the right with opacification of right lung (*asterisk*). Opacification may very well be due to hypoplasia of lung. Note paucity of bowel gas in abdomen.

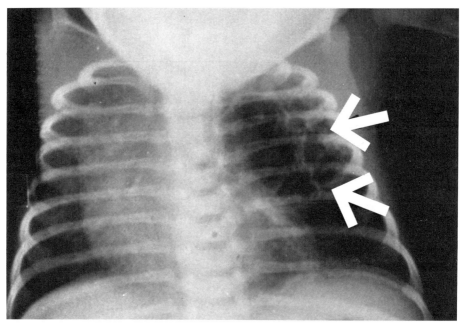

Figure 10–17. Cystic adenomatoid malformation. The malformation is characterized by ill-defined cystic structures (*arrows*).

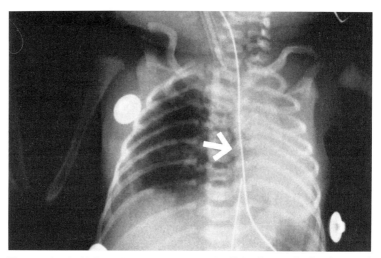

Figure 10–18. Unilateral pulmonary agenesis. This abnormality involves total opacification of left lung with decrease in volume. Note shift of mediastinum to left side (*white arrow*) and closer approximation of ribs on left side compared to right side because of reduced volume on left.

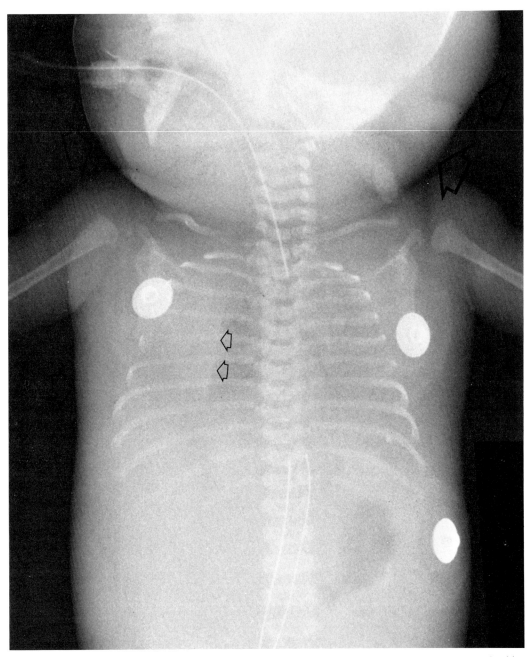

Figure 10–19. Hydrops fetalis. Note diffuse soft-tissue edema (*large open arrows*); ascites is characterized by diffuse hazy appearance of abdomen; pleural effusion (*small open arrows*) is on right side.

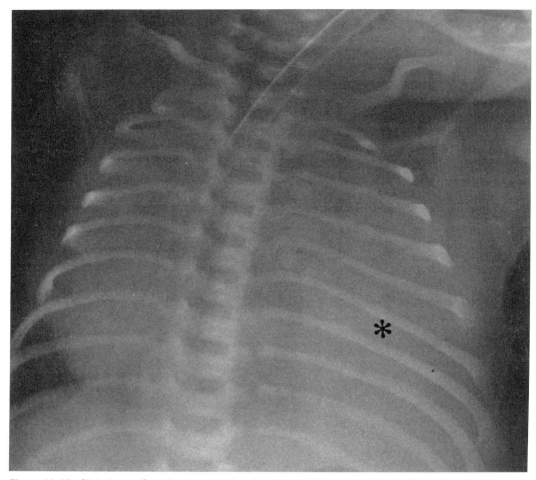

Figure 10–20. Chylothorax. Opacification of left hemithorax is due to massive pleural effusion (*asterisk*).

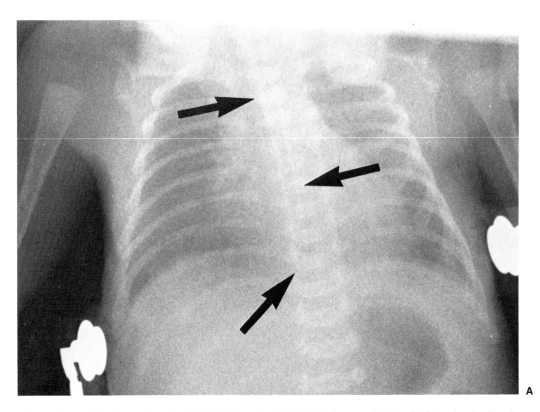

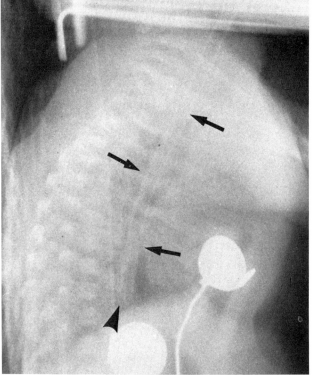

Figure 10–21. Endotracheal tube placement. **A.** Frontal view shows low placement of tube in esophagus (*arrows*). **B.** Lateral film demonstrates posterior position of tube in esophagus (*arrows*). Arrowhead points to endotracheal tube in distal esophagus.

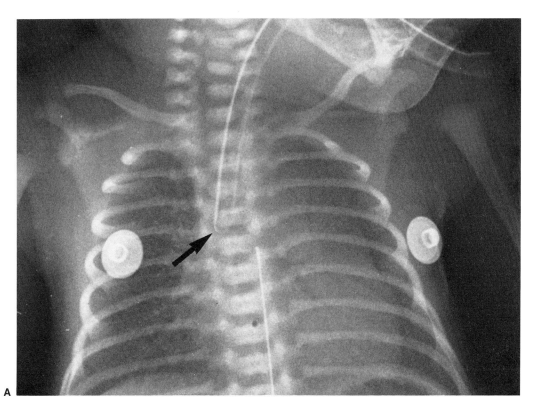

A

Figure 10–22. Endotracheal tube placement. **A.** Tube is malpositioned in right mainstem bronchus (*arrow*). **B.** Endotracheal tube has been withdrawn from low position. High ventilatory pressures have contributed to right pneumothorax (*small white arrows*) and a pneumomediastinum (*large white arrow*); thymus gland is elevated slightly on right, more on left creating spinnaker sign (*asterisks*).

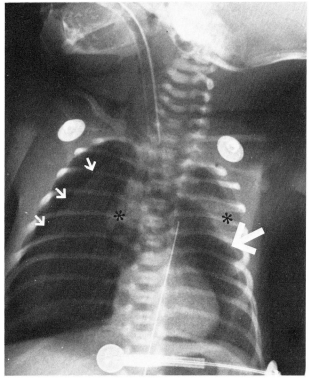

B

Index